P9-DNA-676

the adrenal cortex

A SCOPE® MONOGRAPH

JOHN E. BETHUNE, M.D.
Professor & Chairman, Department of Medicine
University of Southern California School of Medicine
Los Angeles, California

Published by THE UPJOHN COMPANY, *Kalamazoo, Michigan*

Editor / Baird A. Thomas

Library of Congress Card Number 72-79759

S-2890R
Second Edition

Contents

Preface

When I was approached by the Editor of Scope® Publications with the idea of writing a monograph for a pharmaceutical manufacturer my immediate reaction was to say no. However, behaving like the true physician should, my following reaction was to tell him "let me gather some data, examine it and decide". Some time later I received all the monographs in the Scope® series. Needless to say, I was thrilled and excited by the high quality of the script, the bookmaking and above all the unparalleled number and quality of the illustrations. Here was an opportunity to share with my peers many of the patients and materials I had been gathering for years in my endeavors as a teacher and student.

In keeping with the theme of the series I have attempted to present a simplified but comprehensive and up-to-date espousal of the "art" of the adrenal cortex today for the medical student. Some will find certain chapters "stand on their own", to the extent that there is no need for the average medical student to read any single chapter to understand another. The glossary should also help. The chapters on chemistry, physiology and treatment may be boringly detailed—I hope some of the other chapters will turn you on sufficiently to read the rest. To clearly grasp the basic science of the adrenal cortex is an essential to the joy of being able to express to yourself when confronted with a clinical problem—"I understand it." To me, medicine is a hobby from which I can make a living. Without these joys it would just be another job. I simply hope you can get from these pages an understanding that will help you in the same way.

John E. Bethune

1 *2*

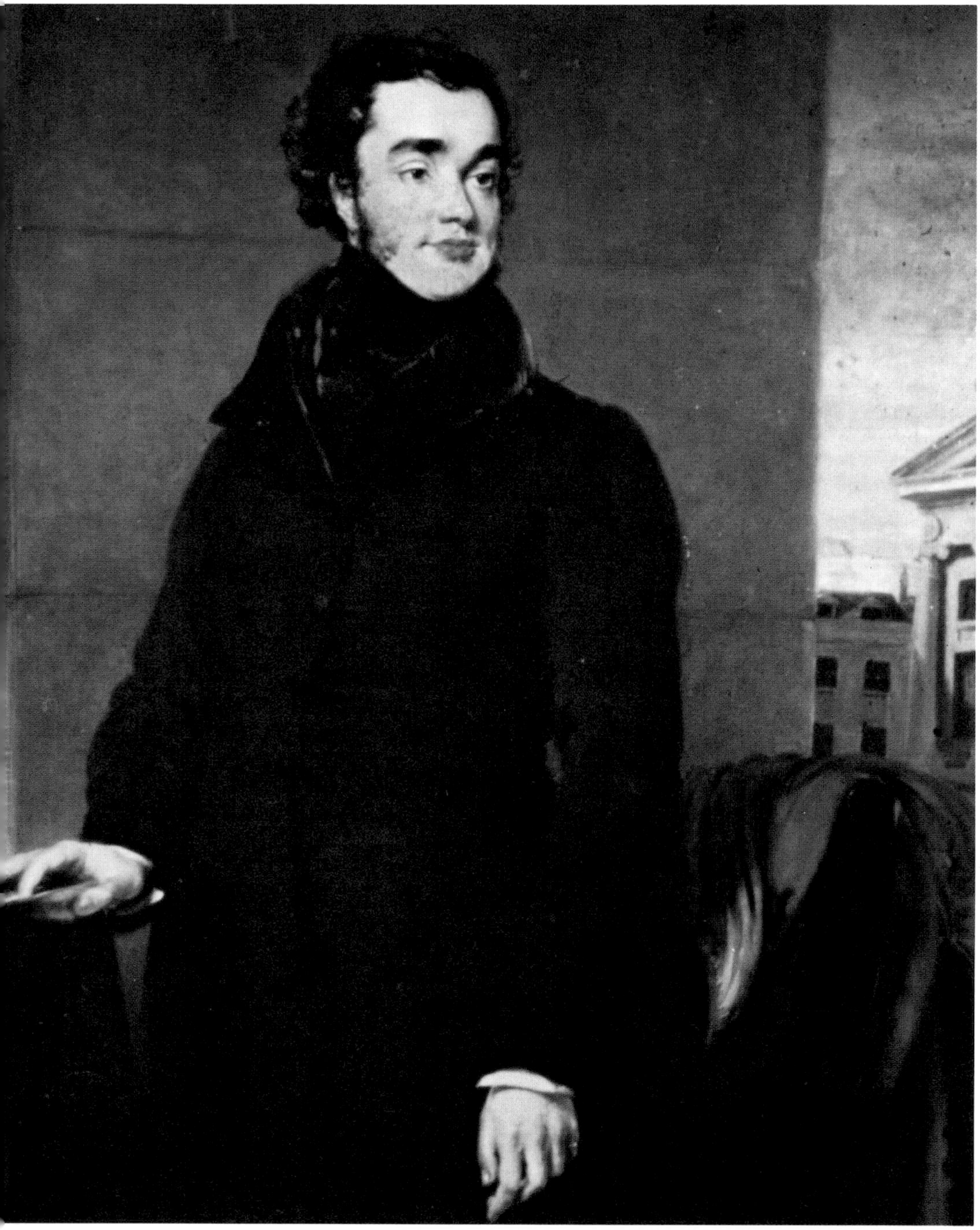

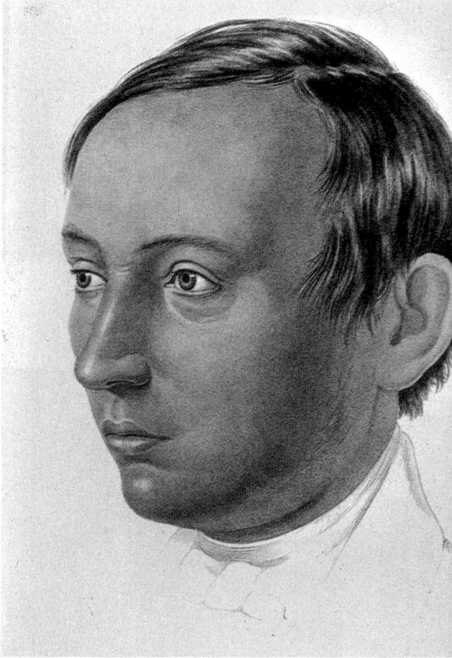

3

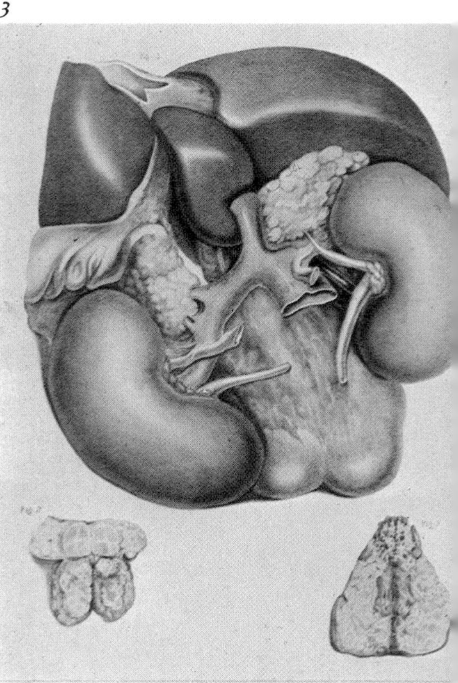

1 Historical Background

"It will hardly be disputed that at the present moment, the functions of the supra-renal capsules, and the influence they exercise in the general economy, are almost or altogether unknown. The large supply of blood which they receive from three separate sources; their numerous nerves, derived immediately from the semilunar ganglia and solar plexus; their early development in the foetus; their unimpaired integrity to the latest period of life; and their peculiar gland-like structure; all point to the performance of some important office: nevertheless, beyond an ill-defined impression, founded on a consideration of their ultimate organization, that, in common with the spleen, thymus and thyroid body, they in some way or other minister to the elaboration of the blood, I am not aware that any modern authority has ventured to assign to them any special function or influence whatever."

Thus, in 1855 did Thomas Addison, in his brief but classic treatise, "On Disease of the Supra Renal Capsules" inaugurate the modern era of clinical adrenal pathophysiology. When you have completed this monograph, return to this quotation from the pen of one of the most eminent physicians of his time. Perhaps it will induce you to read the entire work. In the century since it was written much has been accomplished, yet nothing dwarfs the contribution of this great mind whose powers of observation are so simply and eloquently exposed in this milestone of medical literature.

His clinical depiction of the disease cannot be improved upon. The description of the pigmentation, (beautifully illustrated in color) the weakness, the gastrointestinal symptoms, the feeble pulse and fatal prognosis remain the basic features for a clinical diagnosis.

4

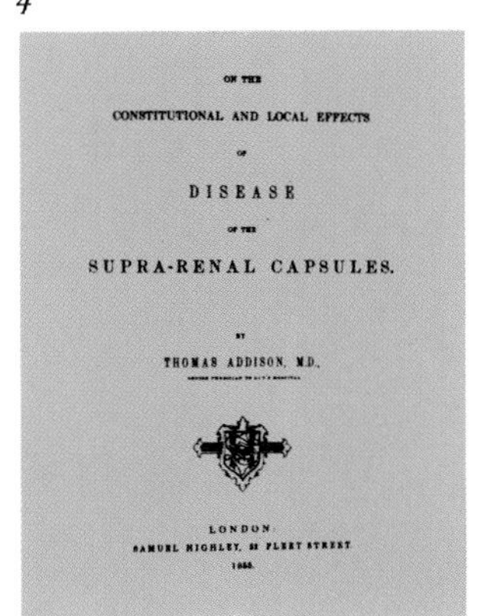

ON THE

CONSTITUTIONAL AND LOCAL EFFECTS

OF

DISEASE

OF THE

SUPRA-RENAL CAPSULES.

BY

THOMAS ADDISON, M.D.

LONDON:

SAMUEL HIGHLEY, 32 FLEET STREET

1855.

Fig. 1 *Thomas Addison. Portrait hanging in the museum of Guy's Hospital, London, England.*

Fig. 2 *Reproduction of Dr. Addison's first patient showing the typical pigmentation of the disease.*

Fig. 3 *Autopsy drawing of patient in Figure 2 showing the caseous lesions of tuberculosis involving the adrenals.*

Fig. 4 *Frontispiece of Addison's classic monograph on adrenal insufficiency.*

A year later Brown-Séquard published a series of experiments showing that the adrenal glands are necessary for life. However, many years of debate followed Addison's work before a clinical syndrome due to disease of the adrenals was generally accepted by the medical community. In 1901 isolation of epinephrine from the adrenal gland was accomplished. It was definitely demonstrated that this hormone was incapable of maintaining life in the adrenalectomized animal, and it therefore became evident that destruction of the adrenal cortex was the cause of Addison's Disease. It was not until Hartman and Brownell and Thorn, as well as Swingle and Pfiffner, independently prepared extracts of adrenal cortex that maintained the life of adrenalectomized animals, that this was proven. Hartman gave the name "cortin" to this active principle. These studies were a major impetus to the chemical isolation of the "active" principle and to its identification.

Foremost among these researchers were E. C. Kendall, J. J. Pfiffner and O. Wintersteiner in the United States and T. Reichstein in Switzerland. In 1936 the first crystalline product with biologic activity was isolated by Kendall's group and designated Compound E (later called cortisone). The same steroid was designated Compound F by Wintersteiner and Pfiffner, and Compound Fa by Reichstein. Thus began a confusing terminology only recently clarified. (See Chapter 3)

The structure of several steroids was rapidly elucidated and the first synthetic adrenocortical steroid 11-desoxycorticosterone was synthesized by Reichstein's group in 1937. It was not until 1943 that the first 11-oxy-steroid, 11-dehydrocorticosterone (Compound A) was synthesized by Reichstein. It was, however, a disappointing steroid for it was not useful in the treatment of Addison's Disease.

In 1946 Sarett produced a partial synthesis of Compound E and by mid-1948 this compound, now named cortisone, was being synthesized in gram quantities. It was effective in the management of Addison's disease.

In the meantime Dr. Philip Hench at the Mayo Clinic reasoned from observations on the effects of pregnancy and jaundice on rheumatoid arthritis that steroids might be a useful treatment. The first trial of some of Kendall's cortisone that had been sitting on a shelf, unused, was begun in September 1948. The results were dramatic. Thus began the era that has seen these powerful therapeutic tools increase in use until they now are one of the most frequently prescribed drugs.

Overdosage of patients with this hormone was quickly seen to resemble the disease described in a group of patients by Dr. Harvey Cushing in 1932 as due to Pituitary Basophilism. Hyperadrenocortisonism and Cushing's Syndrome became synonymous. Dr. Cushing first described the disease that bears his name in a paper on a patient, Minnie G. that first appeared in 1912. He was able by 1932, the date of his definitive paper on the subject, to gather data on an additional eleven patients. The conflict between a pituitary and adrenal origin of this syndrome, not yet completely resolved, began with this paper.

The end was not in sight. The chemists had isolated at least twenty-six different steroids from adrenal cortical extracts. Some with significant biologic activity were yet to be found.

Thus, Dr. James Tait and Miss Sylvia Simpson, in England, (later Dr. & Mrs. Tait) crystallized a new potent mineralocorticoid from the amorphous extract of the adrenal cortex. The crystalline material was sent to Dr. Reichstein in Switzerland, who found on chemical analysis that it had a most unusual structure—an aldohyde group was present on carbon atom 18. It was named aldosterone. Their discovery had earlier been suggested by Dr. John Leutscher of Stanford University from his finding of a potent sodium retaining factor in the urine of patients with edema.

Only a year later, Dr. Jerome Conn dramatically described a syndrome compatible with what would be expected from an excess secretion of this newly discovered and synthesized mineralocorticoid. The exigencies of war had primed Dr. Conn's mind to recognize this syndrome. During World War Two he had been assigned to study heat acclimatization, a problem encountered by soldiers in the South Pacific. It was found that heat decreased the sweat sodium to low concentrations, a condition which was produced by the injection of the first synthesized and only available steroid, desoxycorticosterone acetate. When he saw a patient whose biological findings and symptoms suggested similarities to desoxycorticosterone treatment, it seemed clear to Dr. Conn that excess aldosterone was being made by the adrenal. At exploratory surgery a tumor was found in the left adrenal gland. It was removed and the patient was cured. Conn's Syndrome, as it quickly became known, was born.

Since then many researchers have added to the knowledge of the adrenal gland, its hormones, its pharmacology and its control. Yet, much remains to be discovered. The tale of the adrenal cortex is far from ended.

Fig. 5 *Dr. Harvey Cushing. Painted by Mrs. Cleveland Page when Dr. Cushing was 62 years of age. Portrait hanging in the Peter Bent Brigham Hospital, Boston, MA (detail)*

Fig. 6 *Minnie G., the first patient seen by Dr. Cushing, showing obvious features of the syndrome bearing his name.*

Fig. 7 *Dr. Jerome Conn, Professor of Medicine at the University of Michigan, Michigan Medical Center, Ann Arbor, MI.*

Fig. 8 *Marjorie W., the first patient seen by Dr. Conn. Her hypertension and hypokalemia was cured by removal of an aldosterone producing adenoma of the left adrenal gland.*

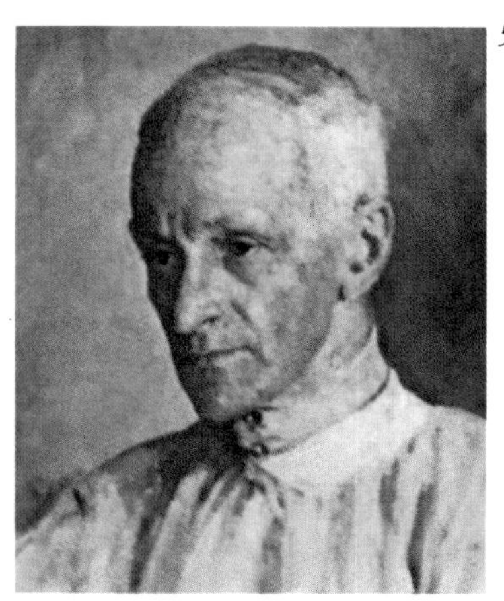

5

Cushing's Syndrome

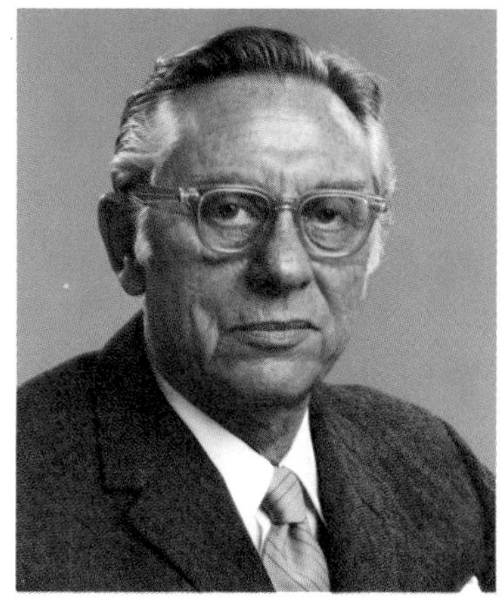

7

Conn's Syndrome

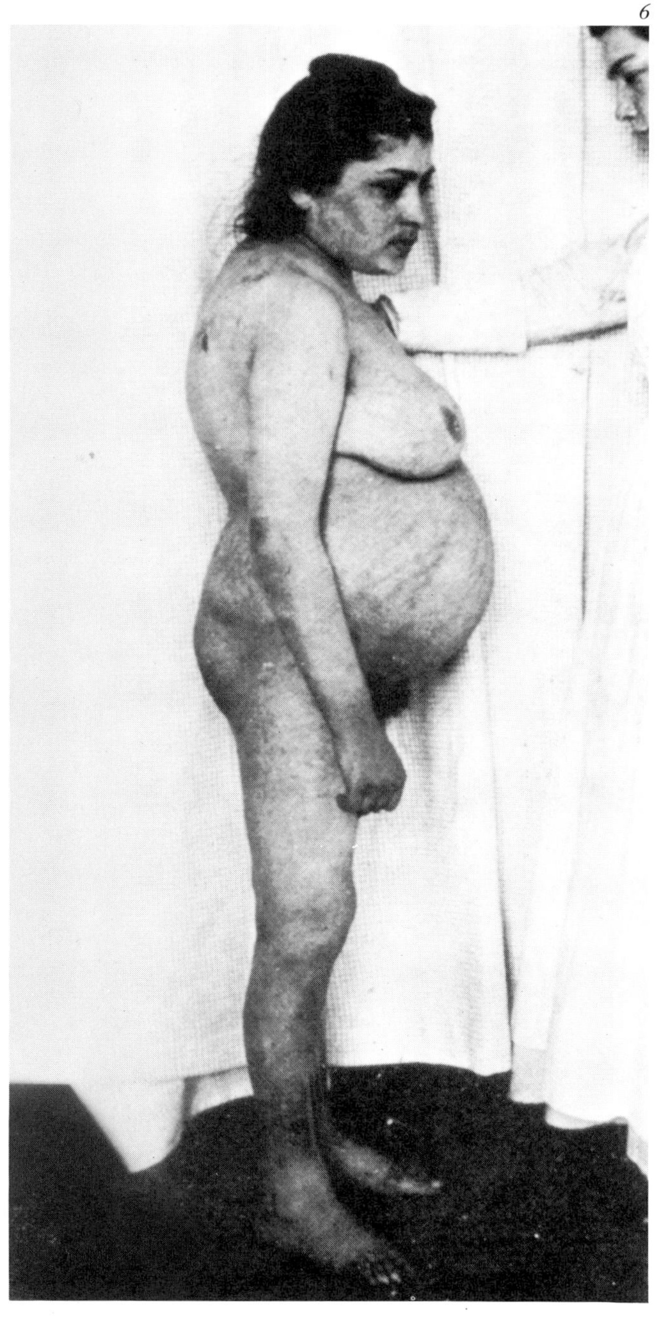

6

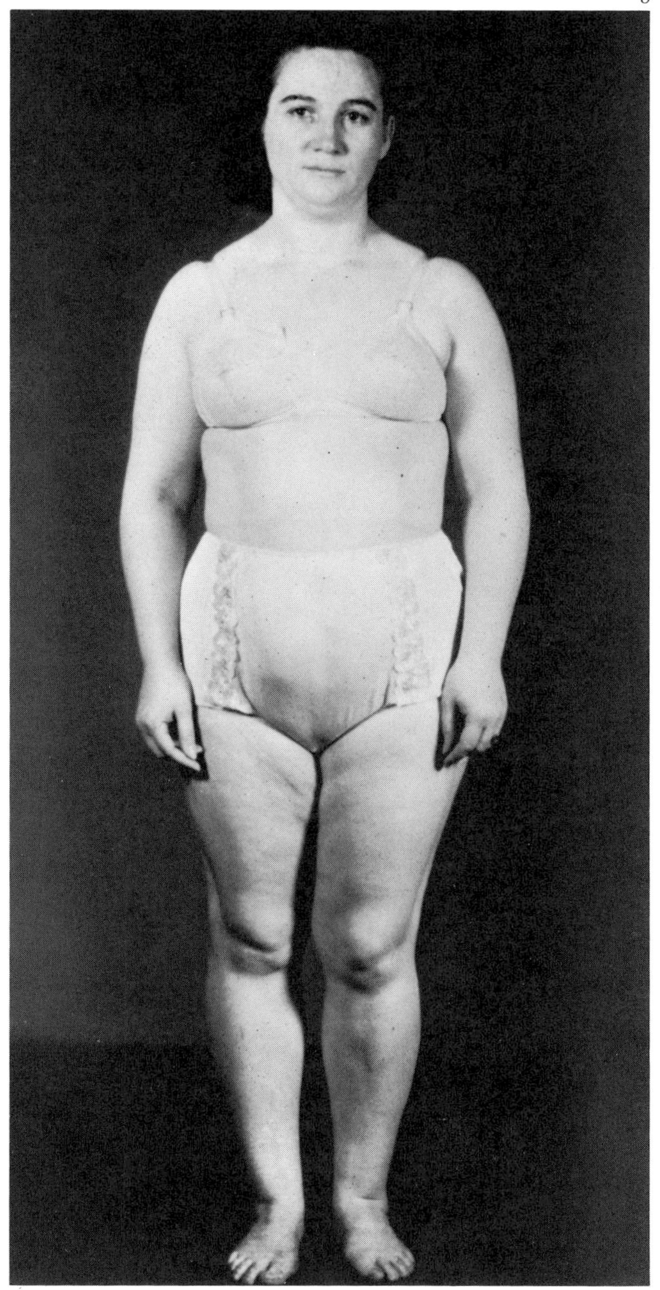

8

2 Fetal Development

The human adrenal gland is considerably different from that of lower mammalian species both in its embryology and its anatomy. Developmentally, the cortex and medulla originate from separate primordia and in many species remain as separate organs. The cortex, arising from mesenchymal primordia in the genital ridge of the embryo, often migrates with this tissue and consequently aberrant adrenal cortex and medulla can extend from the mediastinum to the scrotum. *(Fig. 9)*

The primates are unique in possessing during fetal life an unusually wide cortical zone of large ovoid functional cells. The fetal adrenal gland is as large or larger than the normal adult gland, and in relation to fetal size, it is immense. *(Fig. 10)* It is almost as large at term as the fetal kidney. This human fetal cortex has become confused with the "X-zone" of the mouse adrenal cortex and is sometimes mistakenly called the "X-zone." For years the function of the fetal zone was a mystery. Recent research in several centers has produced strong evidence that the fetal zone produces a well known steroid, dehydroepiandrosterone sulphate (DHAS) which is transported to the placenta and used as a precursor for the production of estrogens necessary for the maintenance of normal pregnancy. The initial clue to this discovery arose from knowledge that anencephalic fetuses (lacking a pituitary gland) were born with atrophy of the fetal zone and the urinary estrogen excretion rates of their mothers was low. The need for this "fetal-placental unit" is lost at birth and the fetal zone disappears rapidly thereafter. The fetal zone cells become indistinct and vascular engorgement occurs to such a degree that the cortex may appear to the unwary pathologist as abnormal adrenal hemorrhage. Should no other cause of death be found, the death of an infant at that age may mistakenly be attributed to "hemorrhage of the adrenals." This "hemorrhage" is physiologic.

Morphology

The combined weight of human adrenal glands obtained from victims of sudden death or at surgery without the stress of preceeding long term illness is 7 to 9 grams. At autopsy in patients dying of long term illness, weights up to 12 grams are not unusual. The right gland is triangular in shape, the left is more pear-shaped. Too frequently descriptions of the adrenal cortex have been based on concepts learned from laboratory animals in which the adrenal gland is likened to an egg, the yolk (medulla) completely enveloped by the white (cortex). This concept is clearly untrue in man although surprisingly this information has only been recently obtained. In fact, in the human, the medulla occupies only a portion of the gland, the head and body, while the tail is all cortex. *(Fig. 11)* The anterior aspect of both glands is flat while the posterior aspect of both is ridged into a crest flanked by two wings, the alae.

Blood Supply

For its size, the adrenal is one of the most vascular organs in the body. The blood flow of a normal adult

Fig. 9 *Location of sites where aberrant adrenal tissue has been found.*

Fig. 10 *Relative size of adrenal cortex and medulla* in utero, *infancy, and adolescence.*

9

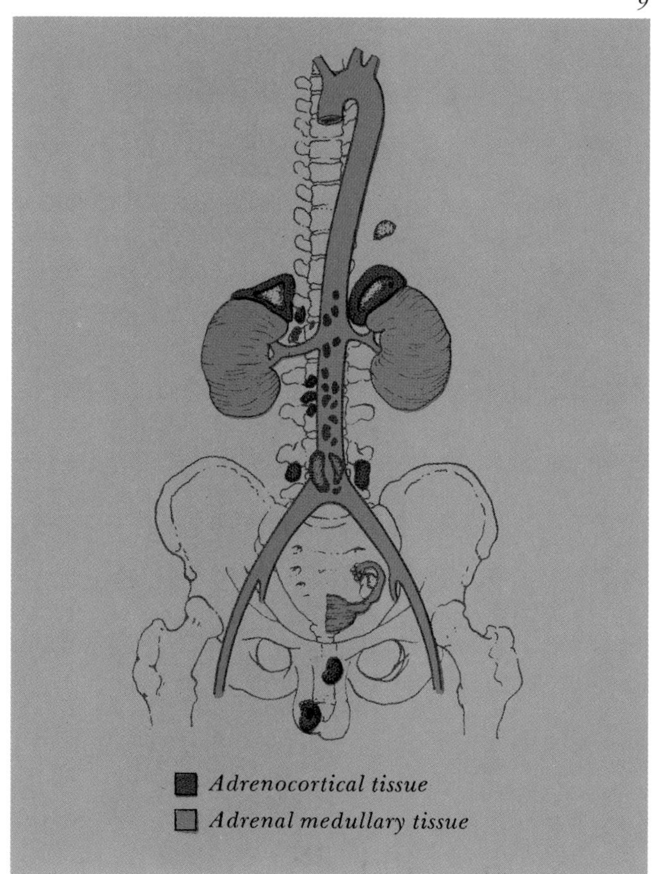

10

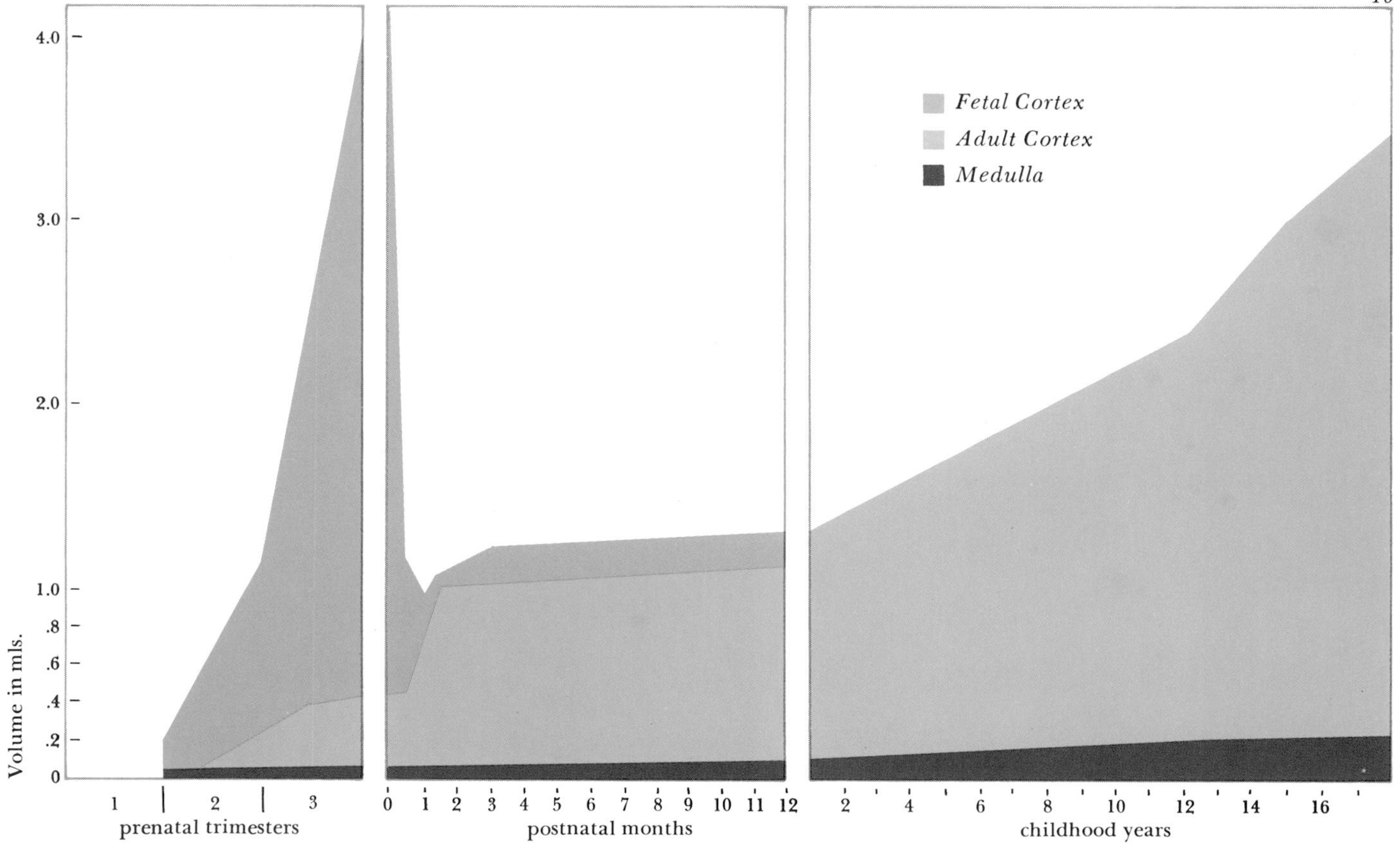

human adrenal gland has been estimated to be 5 ml per minute. Conceptually this makes sense. The hormones of the human adrenal gland are essential to life in stress or shock. When systemic blood pressure and flow is lowered by loss of blood or trauma, the adrenal cortex must maintain an adequate circulation and release of hormones. Its circulatory anatomy is designed to accomplish this. Twenty to fifty arterial branches arise from three major sources to supply each gland. *(Fig. 12)* Their number and pattern is extremely variable, almost no two persons having a similar arterial supply. This situation unfortunately makes adrenal arteriographic visualization difficult and haphazard. *(Fig. 13)* These arterial branches spread over the adrenal capsule, pierce it and organize into a subcapsular plexus at the cortico-medullary junction. There they form a type of portal circulation which then drains by relatively few veins through the medulla to the central vein. There also exists a channel of emissary veins allowing blood to flow back to the glandular surface. The walls of the central vein contain a longitudinal ridge of smooth muscle fibers which has been suggested to con-

11

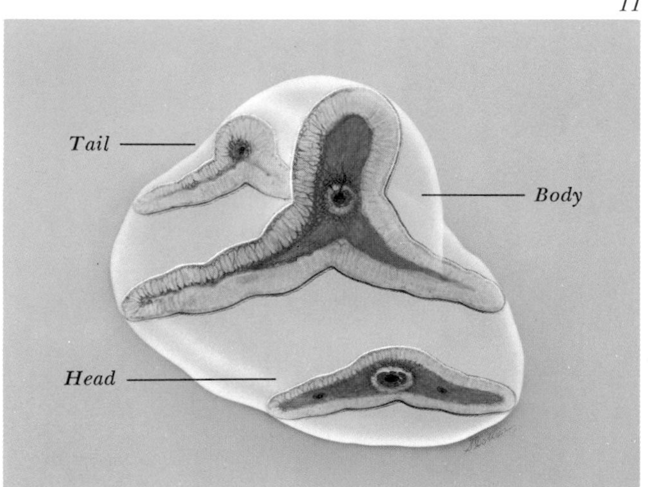

12

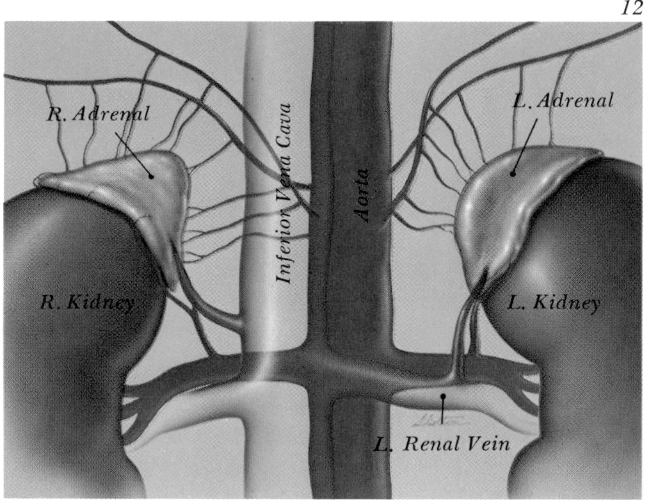

13

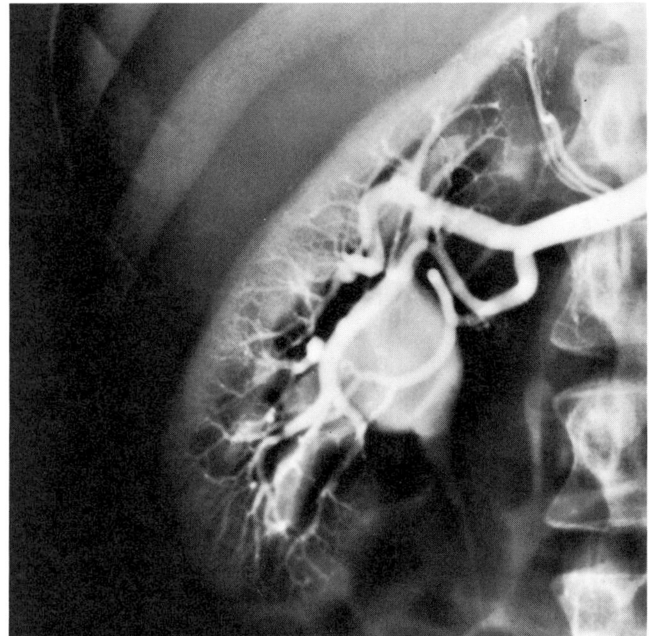
a

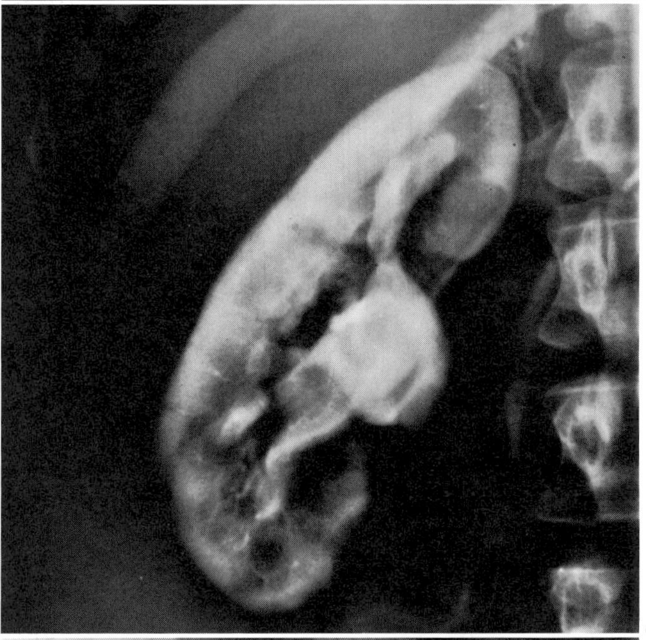
b

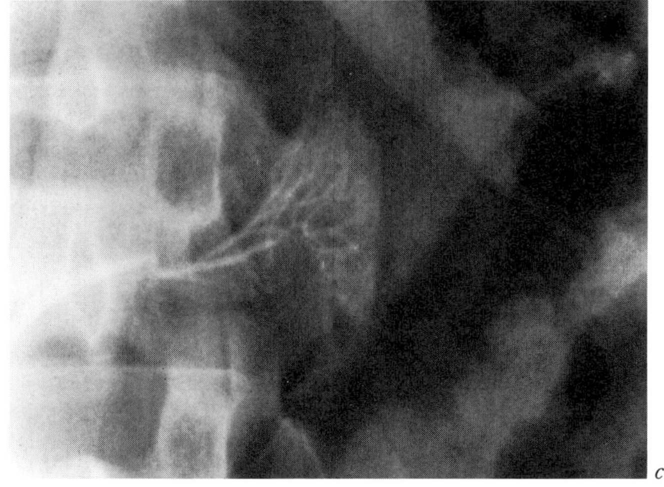
c

stitute a mechanism for producing intermittent stagnation of blood in the juxtaglomerular sinuses thereby exposing the cells of the fasciculata and reticularis more thoroughly to ACTH. Fortunately venous drainage of both adrenals is remarkably constant and through a single central vein. *(Fig. 14)* This vein regularly empties into the renal vein on the left and on the right directly into the inferior vena cava. Thus, collection of the venous effluent draining the glands, and the retrograde infusion of X-ray contrast media into the veins can be readily performed by a skilled radiologist. The use of this procedure—adrenal venography—has greatly facilitated the diagnosis of adrenal cortical adenomas producing Cushing's and Conn's syndromes, as well as confirming the diagnosis of pheochromocytoma. *(Fig. 15)*

Histology

The adrenal cortex was zoned by Arnold in 1866 entirely on the basis of the pattern of the supporting reticulum of the gland without reference to appearance of the parenchymal cells. Subsequent attempts to correlate function and parenchymal cell type to the three zones formulated by Arnold have not been entirely successful. However, the zonation and terms *zona glomerulosa, zona fasciculata* and *zona reticularis* have persisted *(Fig. 16)* and a correlation of the outer zone (glomerulosa) with aldosterone production and the inner zone (fasciculata and reticularis) with glucocorticoid secretion has been established in both man and experimental

Fig. 11 *Human adrenal gland showing relative size of medulla to cortex in the head, body and tail of the gland. Note the vascular lakes at the cortico-medullary junction draining into the large central vein.*

Fig. 12 *Arterial and venous circulation of the human adrenal (Anatomical position). Note the central vein on the left drains into the left renal vein, while the right leads directly into the inferior vena cava.*

Fig. 13a,b *Arteriogram of a normal right kidney and adrenal gland (a). In the venous phase several seconds later (b) the normal right adrenal gland is clearly recognizable by its triangular shape.*

Fig. 13c *Selective left arteriogram of a normal adrenal. The tip of the catheter has been placed in an adrenal artery before the contrast media was injected. In this instance, the entire gland is outlined. Because of the many branches supplying the gland this may not always be the case.*

Fig. 14 *The large central adrenal vein is constant and drains the corticomedullary sinuses and superficial emissary veins. Retrograde infusion of radio-opaque dye through this system is relatively simple.*

Fig. 15 *Adrenal venogram of a normal left adrenal gland produced by retrograde infusion of contrast media through the central vein. The catheter tip can be seen lying in this vein as it enters from the left renal vein.*

14

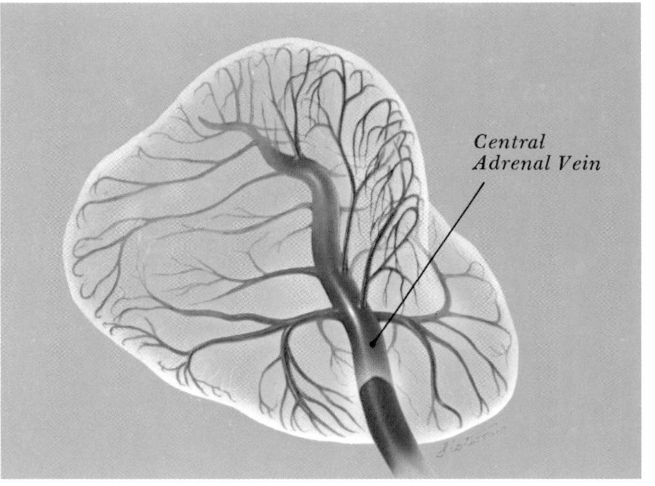

15

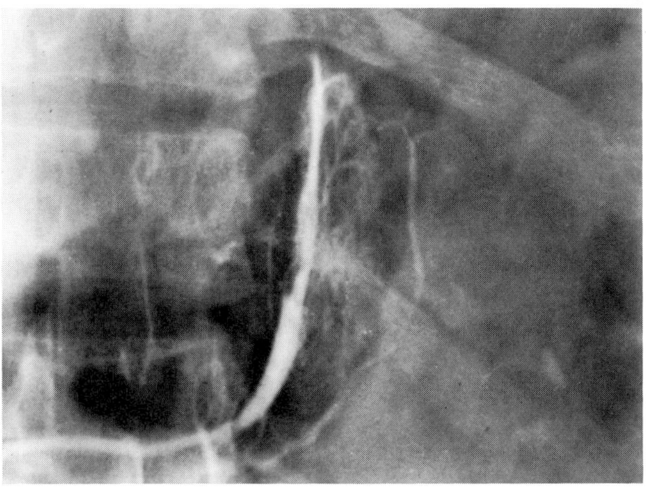

16

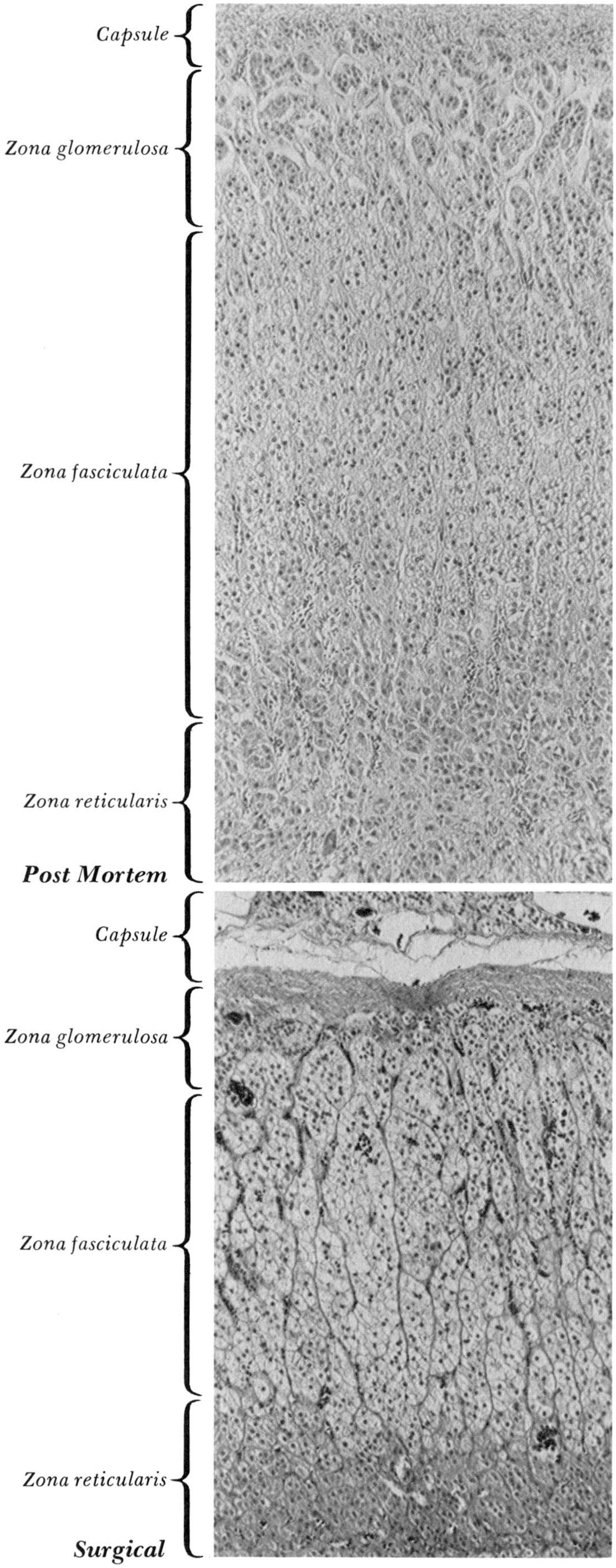

Capsule

Zona glomerulosa

Zona fasciculata

Zona reticularis

Post Mortem

Capsule

Zona glomerulosa

Zona fasciculata

Zona reticularis

Surgical

animals. In general the zona glomerulosa cells have less lipid, are rounded and smaller than those of the zona fasciculata which are polyhedral with a central nucleus, foamy cytoplasm and abundant lipid. The latter type gradually blend into the zona reticularis which contain these cells identical in appearance to those of the zona fasciculata as well as a smaller, darker cell with a deep staining nucleus. In the apparent concern of fitting appearance and function into an ancient stereotyped pattern dictated by a planar pattern of reticulum, the continuous "cord-like" nature of the adrenal cortex has often been overlooked. The adrenal cortex is "liver-like" in the sense that cords of ten to fifteen cells extend from the capsule to the medulla in a continum surrounded by a capillary network—ideally suited for the transport of hormones into and out of cells. *(Fig. 17)*

The ultra-structure of human adrenal cortical cells is similar to other steroid secreting cells of the body in that mitochondria are especially numerous and smooth endoplasmic reticulum (SER) is abundant. The SER is the most prominent feature of all zones and takes the form of a network of anastomosing tubules. Comparative studies of cell content of SER and steroid synthesizing ability have suggested the SER as the site of cholesterol synthesis from acetate. It has long been known that adrenocortical cells are lipid rich. It is highly likely that the walls of the SER are made up of steroid synthesizing enzymes.

Fig. 16a & b *H & E section of two normal adrenal glands collected from two sources x40. The three zones blend indistinctly into one another. 16a)* Post Mortem. *16b)* Surgery. *Chronic stress before death has enlarged the post mortem gland. (see text)*

Fig. 17 *Diagram of the cord-like adrenal cortical cells surrounded by vascular spaces which drain to the sub-cortical plexus creating a form of portal circulation.*

17

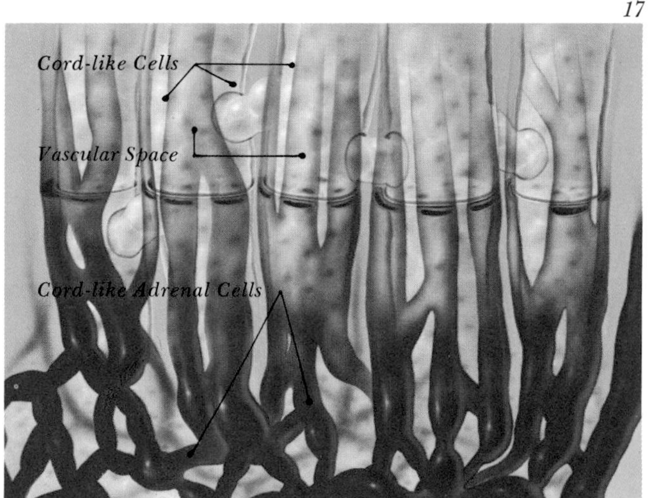

3 Steroid Biochemistry

All adrenocortical hormones are steroids. The term steroid is used to designate those compounds containing a four ring structure, the cyclopentanoperhydrophenanthrene nucleus. *(Fig. 18)* It includes many naturally occuring higher alcohols called sterols such as cholesterol, ergosterol, the glycosides of digitalis and many other substances without alcoholic hydroxyl groups such as estrogens and progesterone.

The terminology for steroids is confusing because of the use of trivial names, chemical names, and different terms for the same thing. Much of this confusion arose in the early days of steroid chemistry. For instance; the most abundantly secreted steroid from the adrenal cortex is commonly known as cortisol. Its chemical name is 11β, 17, 21-trihydroxy, pregn-4-ene-3, 20-dione. Since it is a 17-hydroxy derivitive of corticosterone, it has also been called 17-hydroxycorticosterone; likewise its trivial name is hydrocortisone, implying it is a hydrogenated derivative of cortisone. To further confuse the picture, before its complete structure was known, it was designated Compound M by Reichstein and Compound F by Kendall.

However, the essentials of terminology are relatively simple and a few minutes spent mastering them will be rewarded by an improved understanding of steroid physiology in adrenal disease.

Nomenclature

The basic steroid nucleus, the cyclopentanoperhydrophenanthrene ring, contains seventeen carbon atoms. Each major steroid secreting endocrine organ of the body produces a single major parent compound containing one, two, or four additional carbon atoms to this basic steroid nucleus. It has therefore become steroid shorthand to call those steroids secreted by the

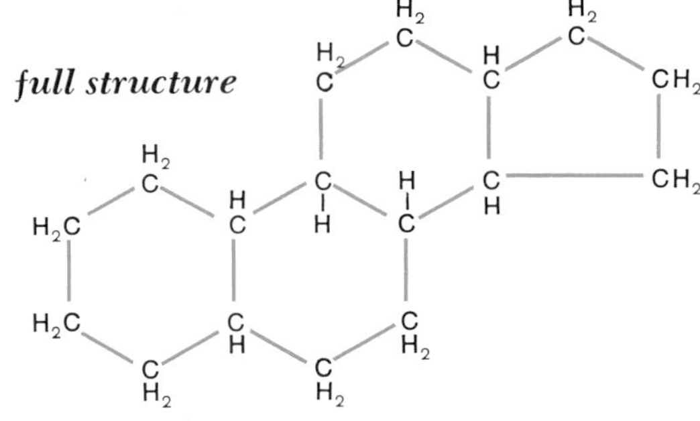

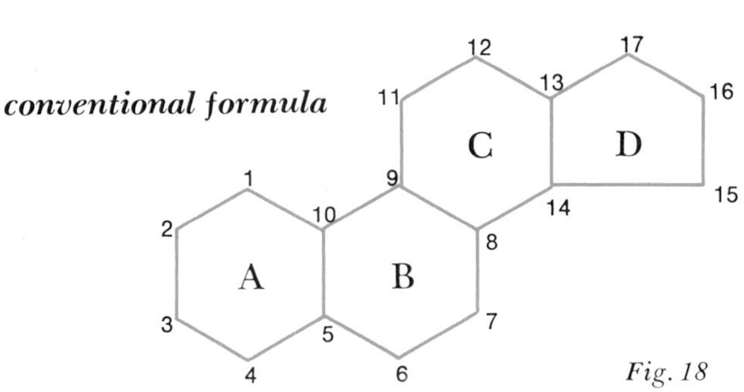

Fig. 18

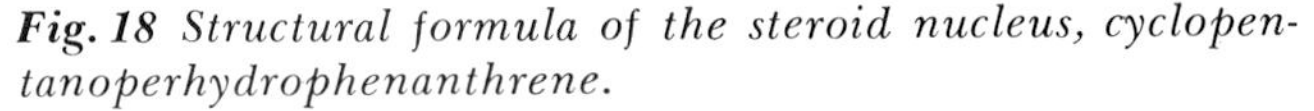
Fig. 18 *Structural formula of the steroid nucleus, cyclopentanoperhydrophenanthrene.*

19

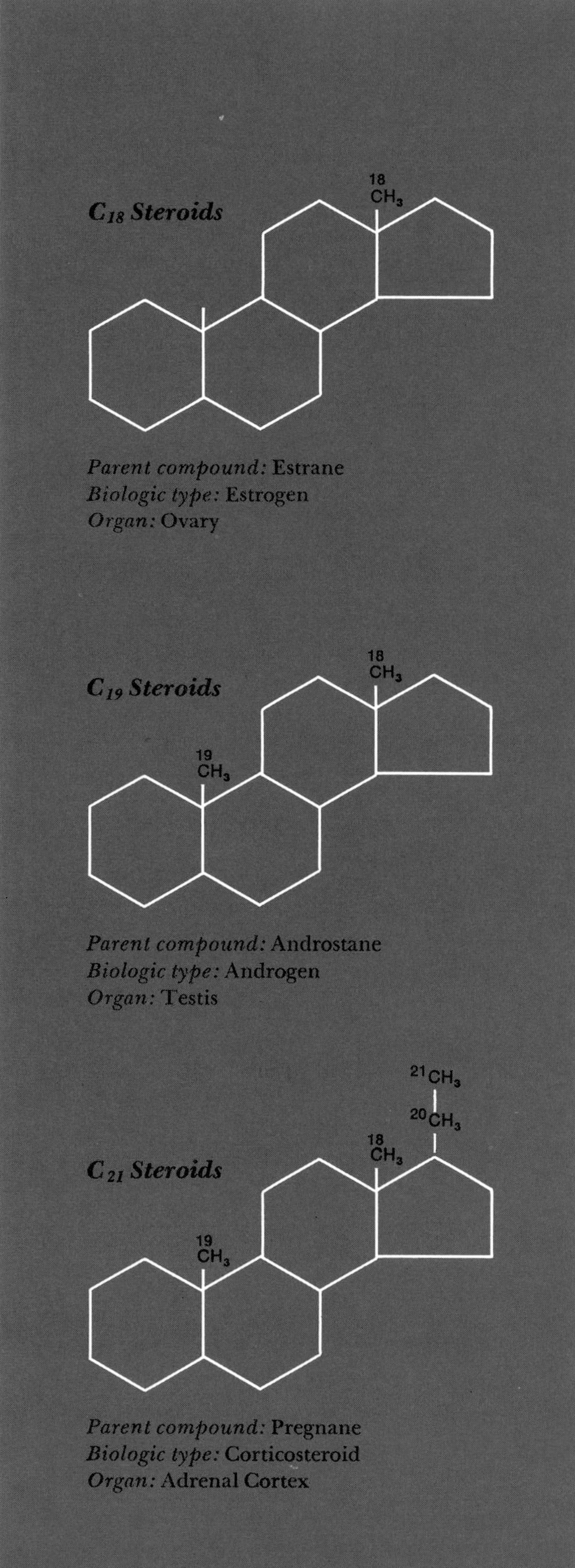

Parent compound: Estrane
Biologic type: Estrogen
Organ: Ovary

Parent compound: Androstane
Biologic type: Androgen
Organ: Testis

Parent compound: Pregnane
Biologic type: Corticosteroid
Organ: Adrenal Cortex

20

prefix	*alteration*	*suffix*
Δ	double (C = C) bond	–ene
Δ	two double (C = C) bonds	–diene
hydroxy	hydroxyl (OH) group	–ol
dihydroxy	2 hydroxyl (OH) groups	–diol
trihydroxy	3 hydroxyl (OH) groups	–triol
keto (or oxo)	carbonyl (C = O) group	–one
	2 carbonyl (C=O) groups	–dione

21

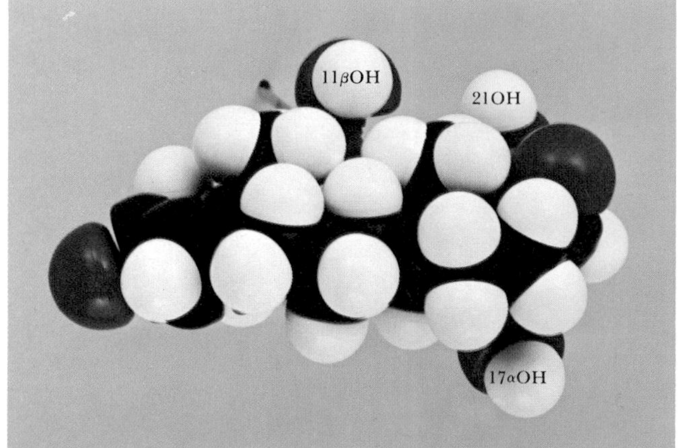

"Ball and stick" rendering of cortisol molecule.

Another view of the above.

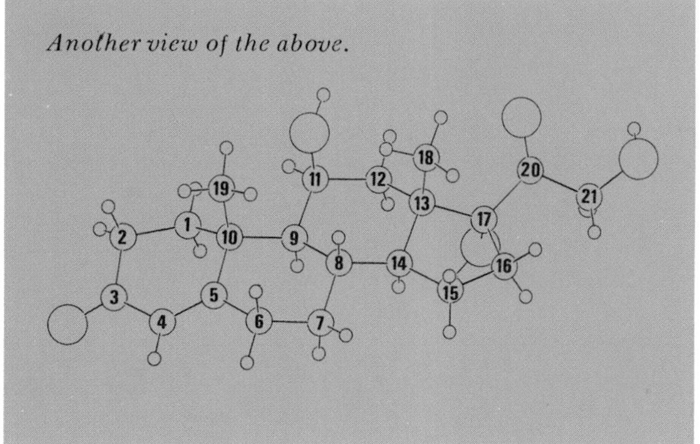

ovaries C_{18} steroids, those secreted by the testis C_{19} steroids, and those secreted by the adrenal cortex C_{21} steroids. *(Fig. 19)* The adrenal cortex also secretes C_{19} steroids as a minor product.

Systematic Names of Steroids

All steroid derivatives from each of the three glands retain the parent compound name modified by prefixes and suffixes designating the type and sight of the alteration to the parent molecule. Only a limited number of alterations can be made. *(Fig. 20)*

By convention only one suffix may be used. The site of a double bond was formerly designated by placing the lower number of the carbon atom adjacent to the double bond symbol $\triangle$, e.g. $\triangle 4$ indicates a double bond between carbon atoms four and five. Recently, the delta symbol has been abandoned in favor of placing the number in the parent compound before the designation of the bond, e.g. ene = 1 double bond, diene = 2 double bonds, etc. The position of a substituted group on the nucleus is indicated by the number of the carbon atom to which it is attached and its spatial arrangement below or above the plane of the nucleus may be designated by a α or β. *(Fig. 21)* Hydroxyl groups are given as prefixes unless they are the only substituents, in which case they are designated as suffixes. Double bonds appear before carbonyl groups as suffixes. To illustrate, the principal human adrenal corticosteroid has a trivial name of cortisol or hydrocortisone, a C_{21} steroid. *(Fig. 22)* The old chemical terminology for this was 11β, 17, 21-trihydroxy $\triangle$4-pregnene-3, 20-dione. In new terminology this is called 11β, 17α, 21-trihydroxy-pregn-4-ene-3, 20-dione. This designates the three hydroxy groups on the 11, 17 and 21 positions; the two carbonyl groups at the 3 and 20 positions and one double bond between the fourth and fifth carbon atom. The most significant hormone secreted by the testis is a C_{19} steroid with the trivial name of testosterone, and is chemically designated Androst—4—ene-17β—ol—3-one. The most significant secretion from the ovary is a C_{18} steroid commonly called estradiol, which has the chemical name estra-1, 3, 5-triene-3, 17β-diol.

Fig. 19 *Parent compounds of the three major groups of biologically active steroids.*

Fig. 20 *Terminology for substitutions to the basic steroid molecule.*

Fig. 21 *Molecular (CPK) model of cortisol. Molecules projecting above the molecular plane are designated β; those below the plane as α; this model shows the 11β hydroxy above the plane and the 17α hydroxy group below the plane of the molecule.*

Fig. 22 *Systematic terms for the three major biologically active steroids of the body.*

Fig. 22

Cortisol

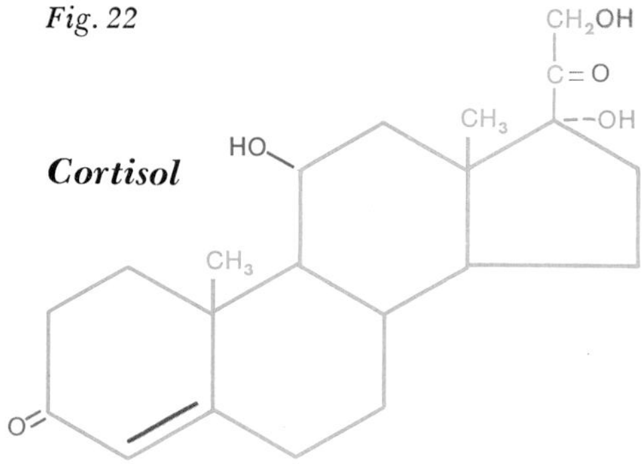

11β, 17α, 21-trihydroxy-pregn-4-ene-3, 20-dione

Testosterone

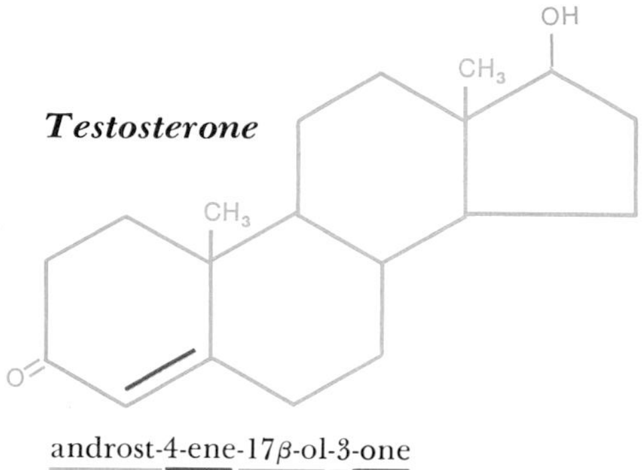

androst-4-ene-17β-ol-3-one

Estradiol

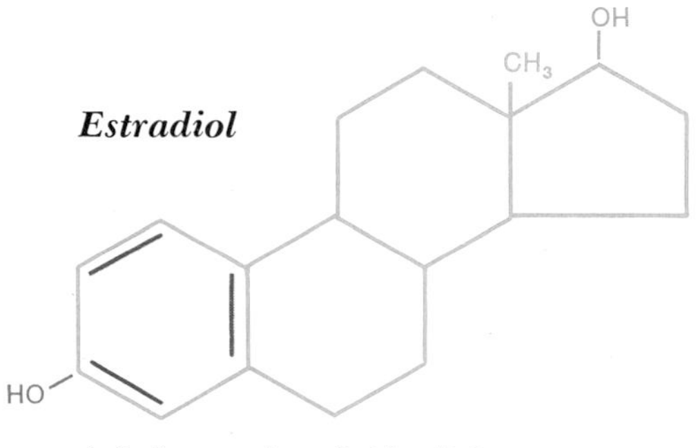

1, 3, 5-estratriene-3, 17β-diol

Fig. 23

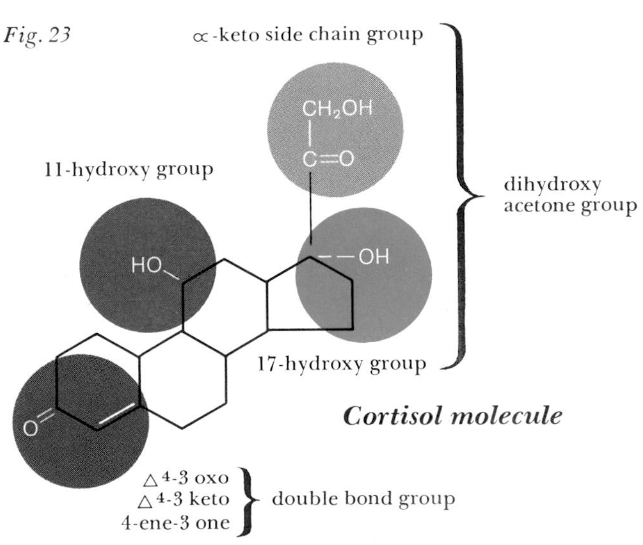

24

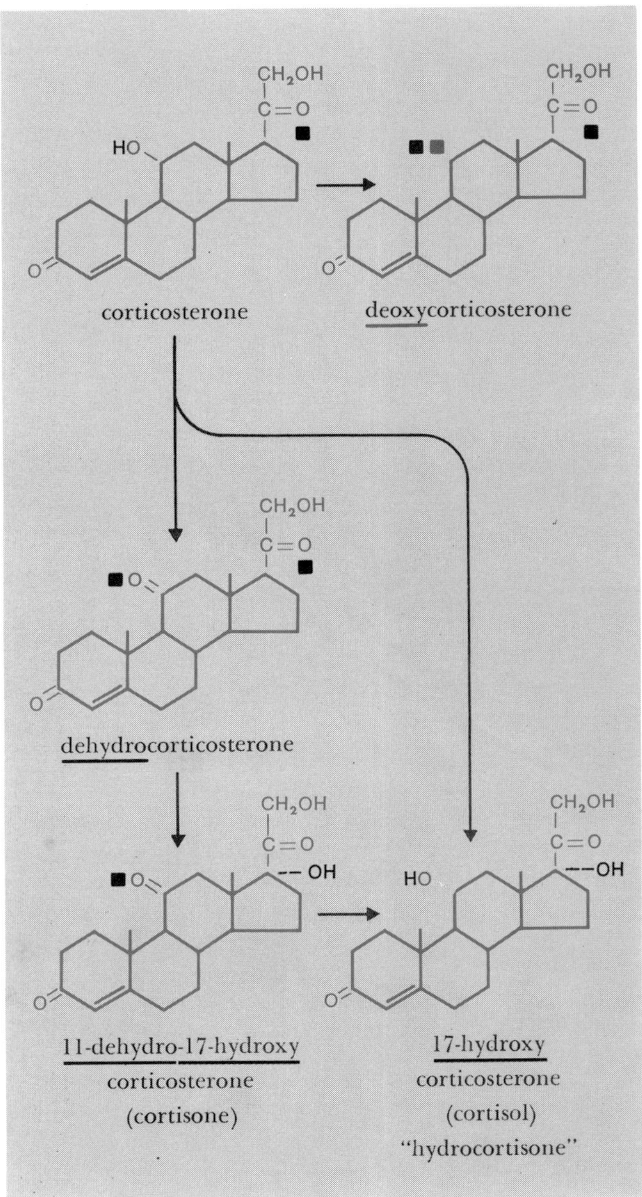

Fig. 23 *The chemical and biologically active groups of the cortisol molecule.*

Fig. 24 *Derivation of trivial names of corticosterone by the addition or deletion of atoms at the 11β and 17α positions. These are not biosynthetic pathways.*

Fig. 25 *Principal adreno-steroids secreted by the human adrenal cortex.*

Fig. 26 *Subcellular road map for cortisol biosynthesis in the zona fasciculata and zona reticularis of the human adrenal.*

25

Class	*Trivial Name*	*Systematic Name*	*Amount Secreted per Day*
Glucocorticoid*	Cortisol	11β,17α,21-trihydroxy pregn-4-ene-3,20,dione	15-30 mg.
	Corticosterone	17α,21-dihydroxy-pregn-4-ene 3,11,20 trione	2-5 mg.
Mineralocorticoid	Aldosterone		50-150 μg.
Androgenic Steroid	Dehydroepiandrosterone (DHEA, DHE, DHA)	3β-OH-androst-5-ene-17-one	15-30 mg.
	△4androstene dione	Androst-4-ene-3,-17,dione	0-10 mg.

*Corticosteroid—A C_{21} steroid with at least 3 oxygen atoms in the molecule. Found in the adrenal gland, blood and urine.

Trivial Names

The systematic nomenclature of steroids is unnecessarily cumbersome for general use and trivial names of the common steroids are used instead. As with systematic nomenclature, prefixes are used to designate relationships of steroids to one another or to alterations made in the parent steroid compound. One of the first steroids used in the treatment of Addison's disease was 11-deoxycorticosterone, suggesting removal of an oxygen atom at the 11 position from the parent compound corticosterone. *(Fig. 23)* Substitution of a hydroxyl group at the 17 position of corticosterone produces 17 hydroxycorticosterone which, since it is a very common steroid, is given the common trivial name of cortisol. *(Fig. 24)* The unique steroid secreted by the outer zone of the adrenal cortex contains an aldehyde group and is simply designated aldosterone.

Over fifty steroids have been isolated from the human adrenal cortex, but only a few are normally secreted into the blood and provide significant biologic activity. They may be classified into three groups as judged by their predominant biologic action. Those adrenal steroids having their main effect on intermediary metabolism are called *glucocorticoids,* those with their main effect on salt and water metabolism are called *mineralocorticoids,* and those with an effect like testosterone are called *adrenal androgens.* They may be thought of as sugar, salt and sex hormones. *(Fig. 25)*

Biosynthesis

Adrenal steroids are synthesized in the cell via cholesterol formation from acetate. In addition, cholesterol is extracted from circulating blood directly into the adrenal synthesizing cell. The common biosynthetic pathway from cholesterol is via pregnenolone, the stem precursor for the three major groups of adrenal steroids. Aldosterone is produced in the glomerulosa while cortisol and adrenal androgens are produced in the zona fasciculata and zona reticularis. Corticosteroid synthesis is a high energy requiring process and is characterized by a complex shuttling back and forth of the steroid between the microsomal endoplasmic reticulum and the mitochondria. The pathway of cortisol synthesis in the intracellular milieu is shown in Figure 26.

The principal chemical reactions which occur in the adrenal are the conversion of pregnenolone to progesterone by two enzyme systems located in the cell microsomes followed by three hydroxylating reactions on specific carbon atoms. These usually occur in consecutive order of 17, 21, 11. The 17 and 21 hydroxylase enzyme systems are associated with microsomes. The 17 hydroxylating system is found in the ovaries and the testis as well as the adrenal cortex but is absent in the adrenal glomerulosa. The 11β hydroxylase system is mitochondrial and limited almost entirely to the adre-

26

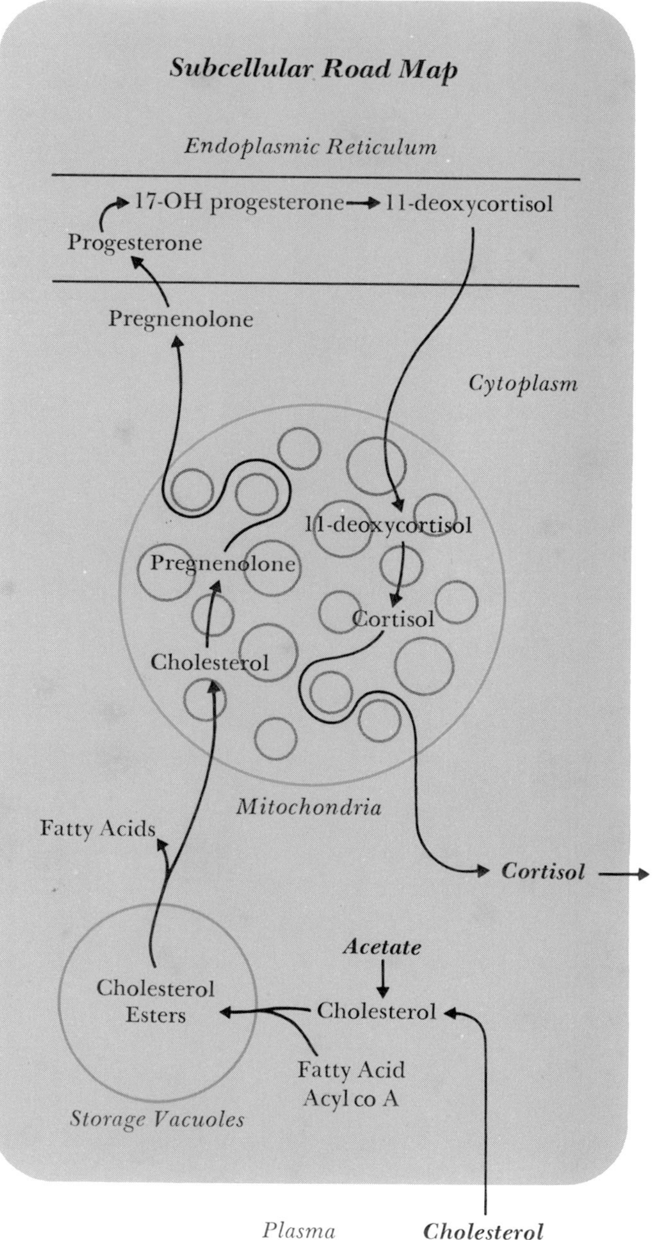

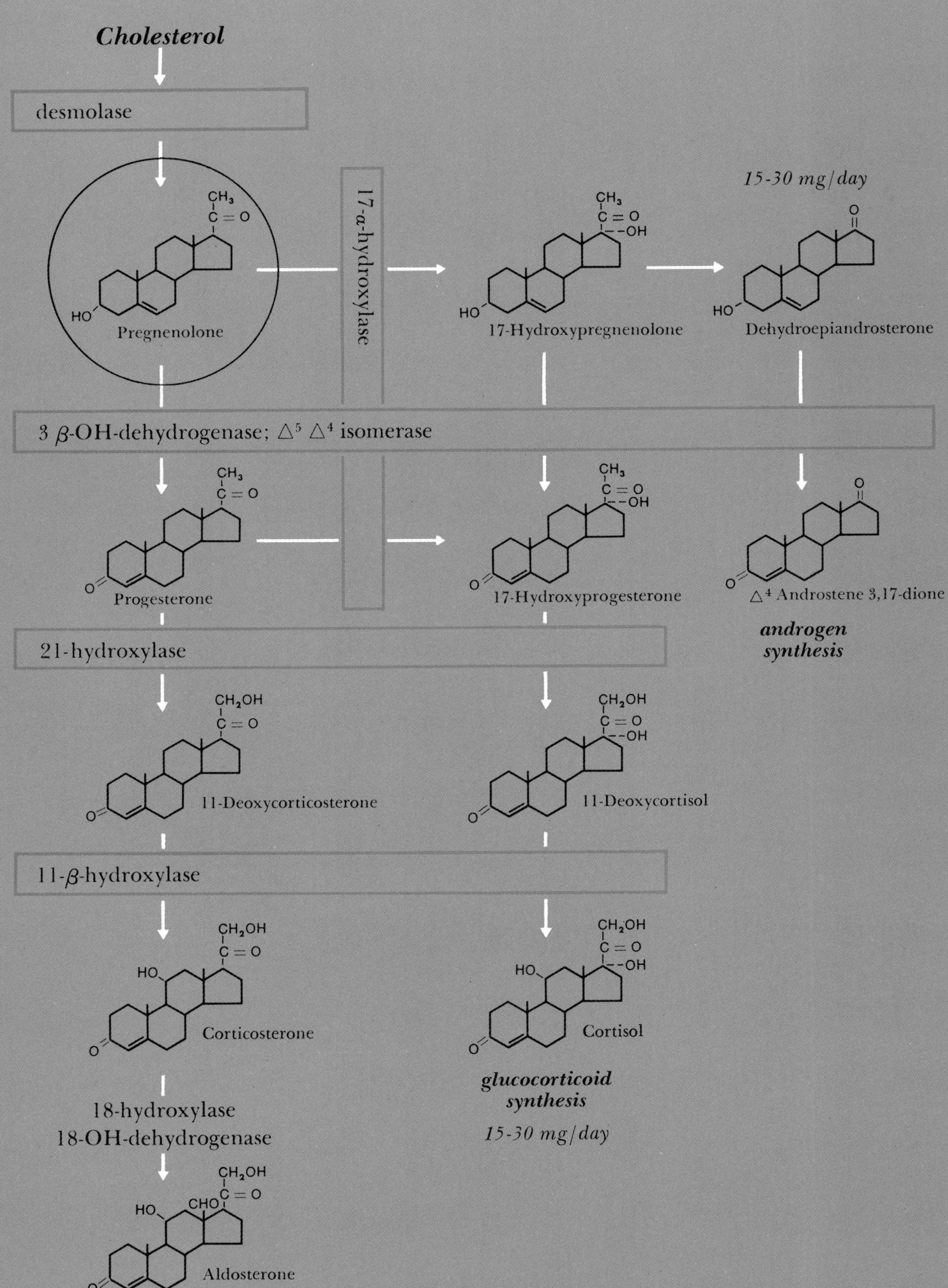

Pathways of Steroid Biosynthesis

Fig. 27

nal gland. This has given rise to the concept that all 11-hydroxy or 11-oxygenated steroids and their metabolites have their origin in the adrenal gland. Therefore the term, 11-oxygenated steroids has been used synonymously with adrenal steroids. Although this convention is generally accepted, it is not entirely true. A fourth hydroxylating system responsible for aldosterone synthesis seems confined to the zona glomerulosa and is responsible for the final production of aldosterone from corticosterone by the reaction shown in Figure 27.

Deficiencies in any one of these enzyme systems should give rise to the production and secretion of abnormal metabolites. In fact deficiencies of most systems have been described and produce recognizable syndromes. These will be briefly discussed later.

Control of Synthesis

Isolated adrenocortical tissues secrete steroids at a low rate and the action of ACTH is required to effect normal secretion and to increase adrenocortical output at times of stress. The precise mechanism by which ACTH induces steroid synthesis and release is unknown. ACTH produces a number of effects on adrenal cortical cells including increased cyclic 3′, 5′,-AMP concentrations; activation of glycolysis and the enzyme phosphofructokinase; increased rate of RNA and protein synthesis and increased conversion of cholesterol and acetate to steroid precursors. It probably initiates these events by acting directly only on the cell membrane, thereby activating adenylcyclase on the inner membrane of the cell wall. *(Fig. 28)* This converts ATP to cyclic 3′, 5′-AMP which then acts as the intracellular second messenger and effects these multiple changes. Those changes seen earliest are secretion of steroids and production of precursors while later and perhaps secondarily, enzyme synthesis is stimulated, increasing the overall capacity of the system to function under a state of prolonged extra need. The release of steroids has been associated with the depletion of ascorbic acid content within the adrenal cortex. To date the exact role of ascorbic acid in the production of steroids following the initial action of ACTH in the adrenal cortex is unknown.

Steroid Transport Systems

Steroids are only sparingly soluble in water. The body has developed methods of solublizing them by binding them to plasma proteins. These act as an efficient transport system and constitute a ready source of preformed steroid in the circulation, available for instant use by cells. Cortisol is reversibly bound in the plasma to two proteins, a specific binding high affinity α_2-globulin called transcortin or corticosteroid binding globulin (CBG) and albumin which has a non-specific low affinity binding for the steroid. At body temperature, 94% of circulating cortisol is bound firmly and 6% is free or very loosely bound to albumin. As free steroid is used up by peripheral tissues, it is directly replaced from this large "protein bound bank," which is replenished by adrenal secretion.

CBG acts as a buffer, insuring a steady and readily available supply of cortisol at the tissues, despite fluctuations in secretion or removal rates. Since all the binding sites on the low capacity, high affinity transcortin are almost completely saturated at normal concentrations of plasma cortisol, a very rapid increase in cortisol secretion from the adrenal cortex quickly floods the system and immediately gives rise to a greater proportionate free cortisol concentration than in the normal state. Therefore, more biologically active free cortisol is available at the cell and incidentally proportionately more free cortisol is filtered at the glomerulus and excreted into the urine.

Globulin bound steroid is *not* biologically active. Pregnancy and estrogen administration greatly increase the amount of CBG in the body, raising the total plasma concentration of cortisol, but not at all, or only very slightly raising the free biologically active fraction. Decreased binding may occur with androgen administration and with some disease states in which the protein is not properly manufactured. Decreased CBG concentration occurs normally in certain families, who

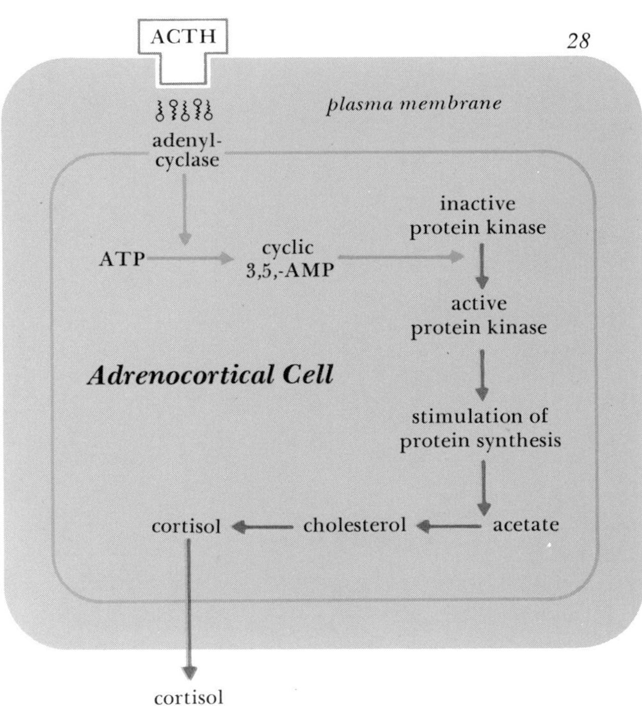

Fig. 27 Three principal pathways of steroid biosynthesis in the adrenal cortex.

Fig. 28 Simplified concept of the molecular events leading to the secretion of cortisol through the action of ACTH.

seem not to suffer from steroid deficiency because free steroid levels remain normal. The free steroid concentration is apparently maintained in a normal range by normal ACTH secretion. Corticosterone is also bound to transcortin, but with less affinity than cortisol. Aldosterone is much less tightly bound and is mainly associated with albumin.

The disappearance rates of cortisol and aldosterone from plasma are closely related to this binding phenomenon. The biological half-life ($T\frac{1}{2}$) of cortisol in the human averages 80 minutes, that for aldosterone 30 minutes. *(Fig. 29)* This biological half-life is a measure of metabolism of the steroid and is very important in assessing potency of various newly synthesized steroids. Since aldosterone is much less bound to plasma proteins than cortisol it is more readily available for metabolism—in fact it is almost completely metabolized to an inactive form in one passage through the liver and it is therefore ineffective as an oral drug. The turnover rate of aldosterone is thus much greater than cortisol and has been estimated to be ten times that of cortisol in the human body. The effect of raising CBG by estrogens or pregnancy is therefore much greater on hydrocortisone than on aldosterone (because of the limited binding capacity of aldosterone). The resultant increase in protein binding in pregnancy leads to a greater increase in half-life of cortisol than of aldosterone.

Metabolism of Adrenal Steroids

Knowledge of the metabolism of cortisol is important to the physician for two reasons:

1. Currently the most frequently used method of assessing adrenal cortical function is by measuring the *metabolites* of cortisol excreted in urine.

2. Synthetic steroids have substitutions or alterations in the molecule which delay or change their method of degradation, thus prolonging and potentiating their effectiveness.

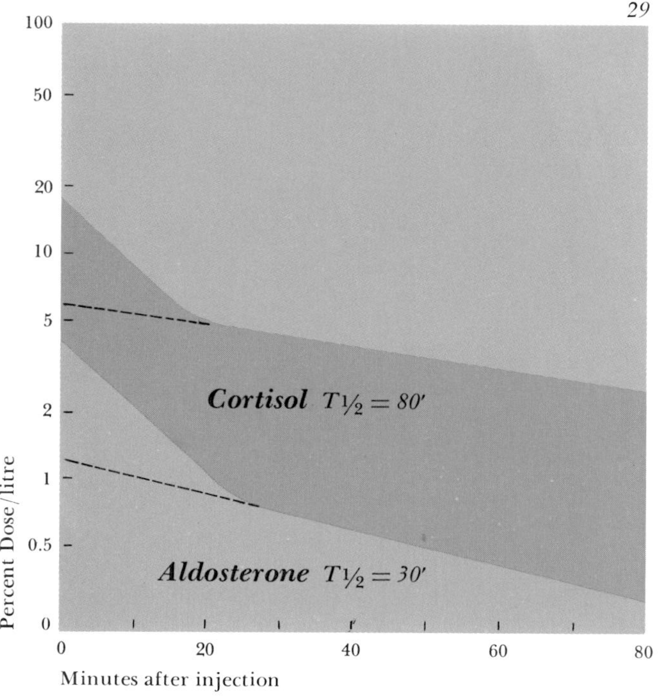

Metabolism of adrenal steroids occurs primarily in the liver. A series of enzymes are found in the liver which are capable of altering the steroid molecule making it both biologically inactive and water soluble. Two main steps are involved in the process:

1. *Reduction* or *side chain removal* of the steroid molecule.

2. *Conjugation* of the altered molecule to glucuronic acid to form a water soluble glucosiduronate, or to sulphate to form water soluble sulphates. The conjugates are water soluble and poorly bound to plasma proteins so they readily pass into the urine.

Cortisol Metabolism

The alterations in the cortisol molecule and its method of disposal are shown in Figure 30. Over 90% of an injected physiologic dose of radioactive 14C labeled cortisol is found in the urine in the succeeding forty-eight hours.

Most of it is excreted in the first twenty-four hours. Less than 1% is found in the urine as free unaltered cortisol. The principal urinary metabolites are tetrahydrocortisol, tetrahydrocortisone, cortols and cortolones. They comprise about 80% of the secreted cortisol while the C_{19} adrenal androgens account for about 5-10% of secreted cortisol.

It is clear that the rate of removal of adrenocortical steroids by the liver together with the adrenal secretory rate and the concentration of CBG determine their plasma concentration in man. In the presence of severe liver disease, the clearance of adrenocortical steroids may be decreased, but since steroid production adjusts to this by negative feedback from plasma cortisol, high blood levels of cortisol do not occur.

Aldosterone Metabolism

Well over 90% of an injected dose of radioactive aldosterone is excreted in the urine in the succeeding forty-eight hours. *(Fig. 31)* 20% to 40% of the material is excreted as a glucosiduronate with the 18-aldehyde group intact (tetrahydroaldosterone). The other major metabolite (5% to 15%) was once erroneously known as the 3-oxo-conjugate, but in fact is now identified as a

Fig. 29 *Disappearance rates of aldosterone and cortisol in normal man.*

Fig. 30 *Metabolism of cortisol in the liver. A significant proportion of cortisone metabolites appear in the urine as products of cortisol metabolism.*

Metabolism of Cortisol in the Liver

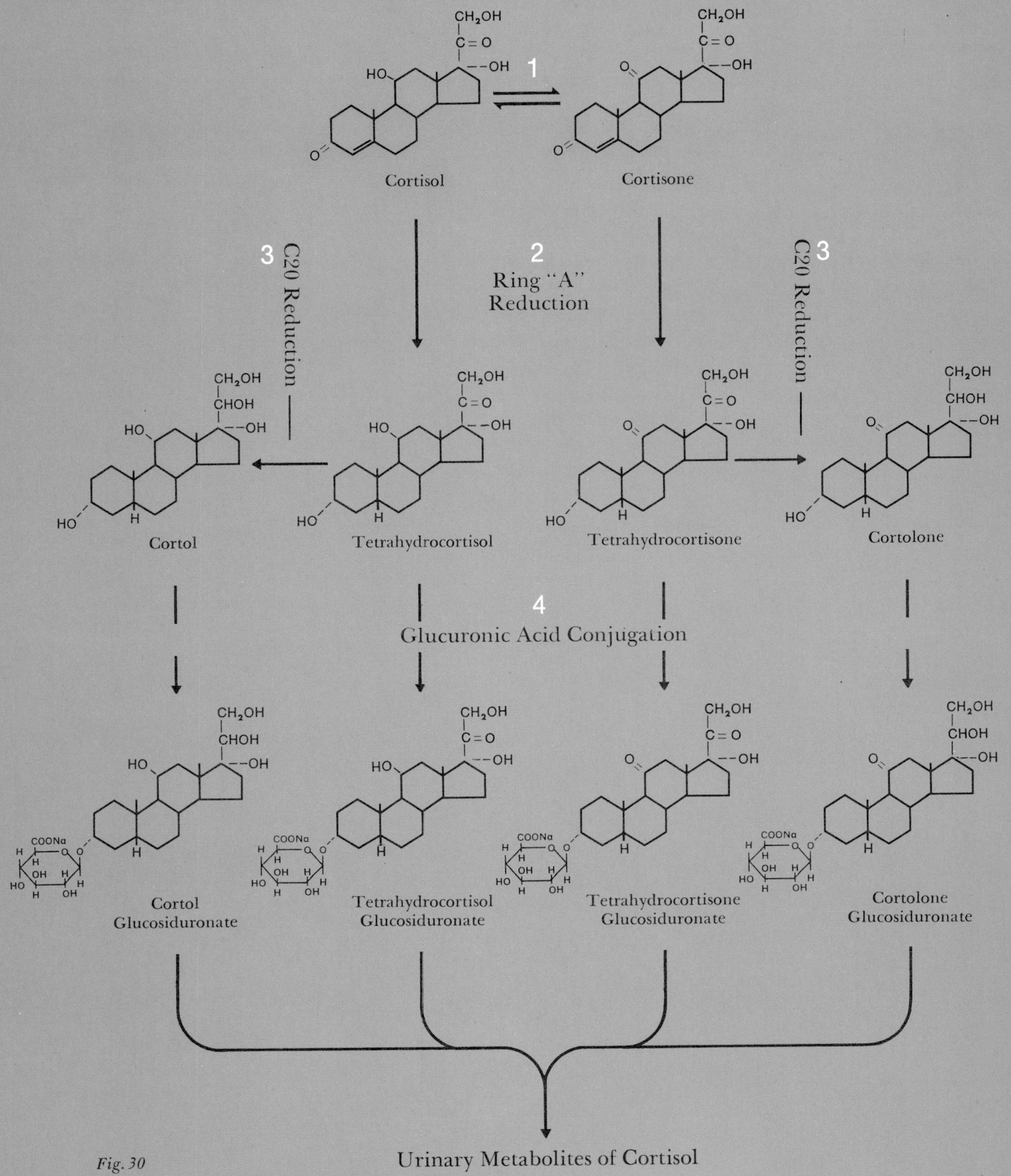

Cortisol ⇌ (1) Cortisone

2 Ring "A" Reduction

3 C20 Reduction

Cortol ← Tetrahydrocortisol

Tetrahydrocortisone → Cortolone

4 Glucuronic Acid Conjugation

Cortol Glucosiduronate

Tetrahydrocortisol Glucosiduronate

Tetrahydrocortisone Glucosiduronate

Cortolone Glucosiduronate

Urinary Metabolites of Cortisol

Fig. 30

conjugate with glucuronic acid at the C_{18} position. The A ring is not reduced in this product. It differs from the tetrahydroaldosterone glucosiduronate in that it is not hydrolysed by the enzyme β-glucuronidase, but is by an environmental pH of 1. It is therefore known as the "acid-labile" conjugate. Methods of measuring aldosterone in urine are usually based on one or the other conjugate and, therefore, estimate only a small fraction of the actually secreted and metabolized aldosterone. Plasma methods of measuring unmetabolized aldosterone are now more popular.

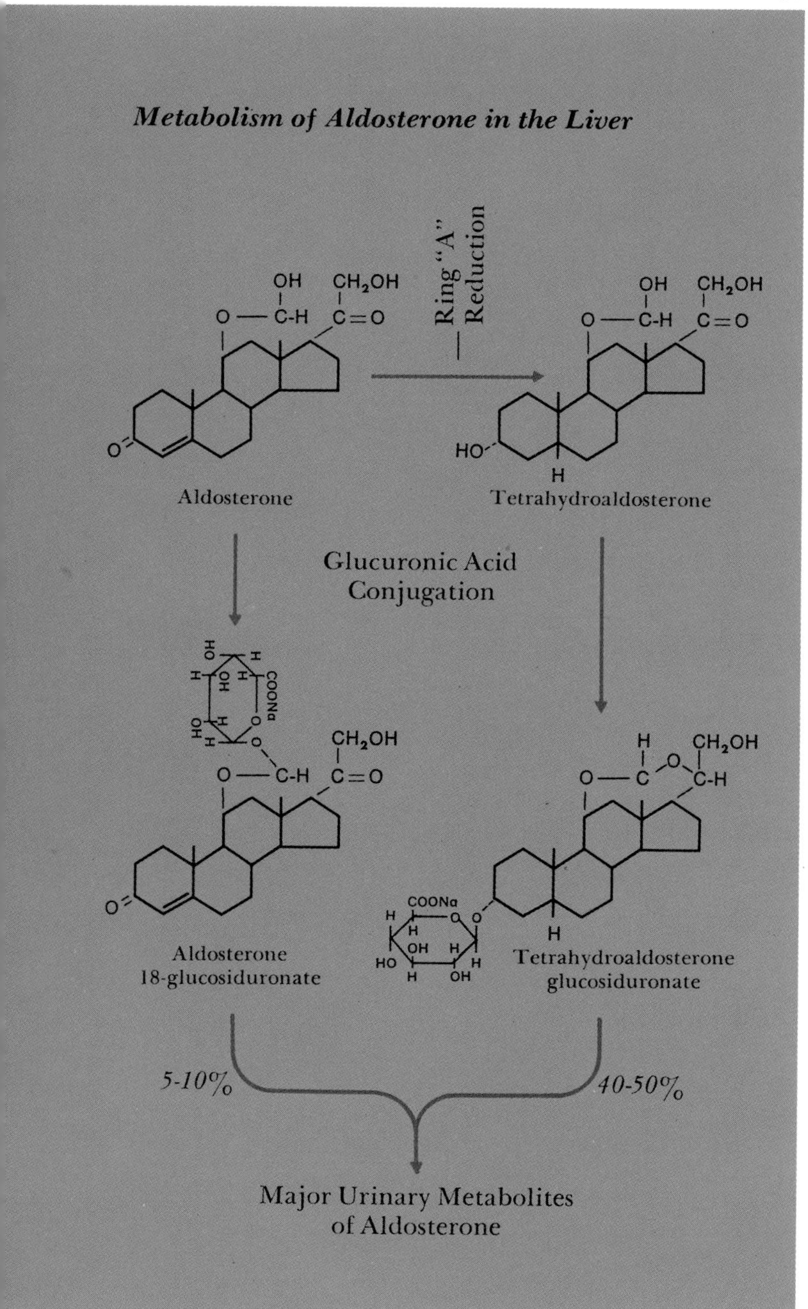

Metabolism of Adrenal Androgens

The adrenal androgens are themselves biologically very weak. They are, however, capable of being converted in many tissues of the body to the potent androgen, testosterone. *(Fig. 32)* They are secreted as C_{19} steroids and eventually excreted primarily as sulphates into the urine. They contribute about two-thirds of the urinary 17-ketosteroids measured by the Zimmermann reaction, the other third in the male is contributed by testicular secretions. The female has one-third lower urinary 17-ketosteroid excretion rates than the male.

Clinical Biochemistry of Adrenal Steroids

Cortisol is the only glucocorticoid circulating normally in human plasma in significant quantities. It is measured by three widely used methods. In all three methods total cortisol concentration is measured, for the plasma extraction procedures used remove both free and protein bound steroid. No method available is sufficiently sensitive to measure free plasma cortisol.

17-Hydroxycorticosteroids (17-OHCS, Porter-Silber chromagens): This accurate, but tedious and costly method measures the yellow chromagen formed from the reaction of a phenylhydrazine-sulphuric acid mixture with those steroids that possess a 17, 21-dihydroxy-20-ketone group. It is thus highly specific for cortisol, its immediate biosynthetic precursor 11-deoxycortisol and the synthetic steroid cortisone. Since the latter two steroids are not normally found in plasma, the Porter-Silber (P-S) method in effect, measures only cortisol. However, drugs may interfere with the reaction.

Fluorescent Cortisol: In the presence of sulphuric acid cortisol fluoresces readily. This fluorescence is given by steroids possessing an 11-hydroxyl group. It is a simple assay to perform and very sensitive, but it is liable to interference by drugs, dirty reaction tubes and to a non-specific fluorescence found in some plasma sam-

31

Fig. 31 *Metabolism of aldosterone in the liver. Two major urinary metabolites are formed.*

Fig. 32 *Metabolism of the major adrenal androgens by the liver.*

ples. It also measures corticosterone, but since so little is present in human plasma no significant interference occurs. This method is not as reliable as either the Porter-Silber method or the Protein Binding Method.

Competitive Protein Binding Cortisol: Cortisol binds specifically to CBG (transcortin). This binding is reversible and cortisol already bound to CBG can be displaced by adding more cortisol to the solution containing the CBG-cortisol complex. If known trace amounts of radioactive cortisol are added to a constant amount of CBG in a test tube, later addition of increasing amounts of "cold" cortisol will displace increasing counts of this "hot" cortisol from the CBG. Measurement of the amount of radioactivity displaced is proportional to the amount of cold cortisol added and a "standard curve" of this may be constructed. If a plasma is extracted to elute the cortisol from the donor's CBG and then continued through this procedure an extremely accurate estimate of cortisol in the plasma sample can be made. *(Fig. 33)* The principle of this "competitive binding" assay is similar to that of radioimmunoassay except that the binder is CBG instead of an antibody. This method is accurate, simple and not interfered with by drugs or non-specific fluorescent material. It is the preferred method today. Specific antibodies to cortisol are already being developed to further improve on this method.

Urinary Steroid Metabolites

Free unconjugated cortisol, as such, is excreted in the urine in amounts too minute to be measured by most available clinical methods. However, extraction of urine before the steroid conjugates are hydrolyzed with acid or enzymes, will yield sufficient "free cortisol" to be measured by the fluorescent or CBG methods used for plasma. Some authorities believe this to be a preferred measure of adrenal secretion as compared to standard methods utilizing estimation of urinary cortisol metabolites formed in the liver. It has not yet been sufficiently used to prove the superiority of urinary free cortisol, and the method is not available in many laboratories. An evaluation of the methods for measuring these cortisol metabolites is therefore still necessary. The major urinary metabolites of cortisol are tetrahydrocortisol and tetrahydrocortisone, both of which contain the 17, 21-dihydroxyketone side chain measured by the Porter-Silber reaction. *(Fig. 34)*

Urinary 17-OHCS (17-hydroxycorticosteroids, Porter-Silber chromogens): Before the Porter-Silber reaction can be applied to urine measurements, the steroid conjugates must be hydrolyzed by strong acid or by a sulfatase and β-glucuronidase to free them from their water soluble glucosiduronates and sulphates so that they can be extracted into lipid solvents. This procedure tends to remove most interfering drugs and combined

32

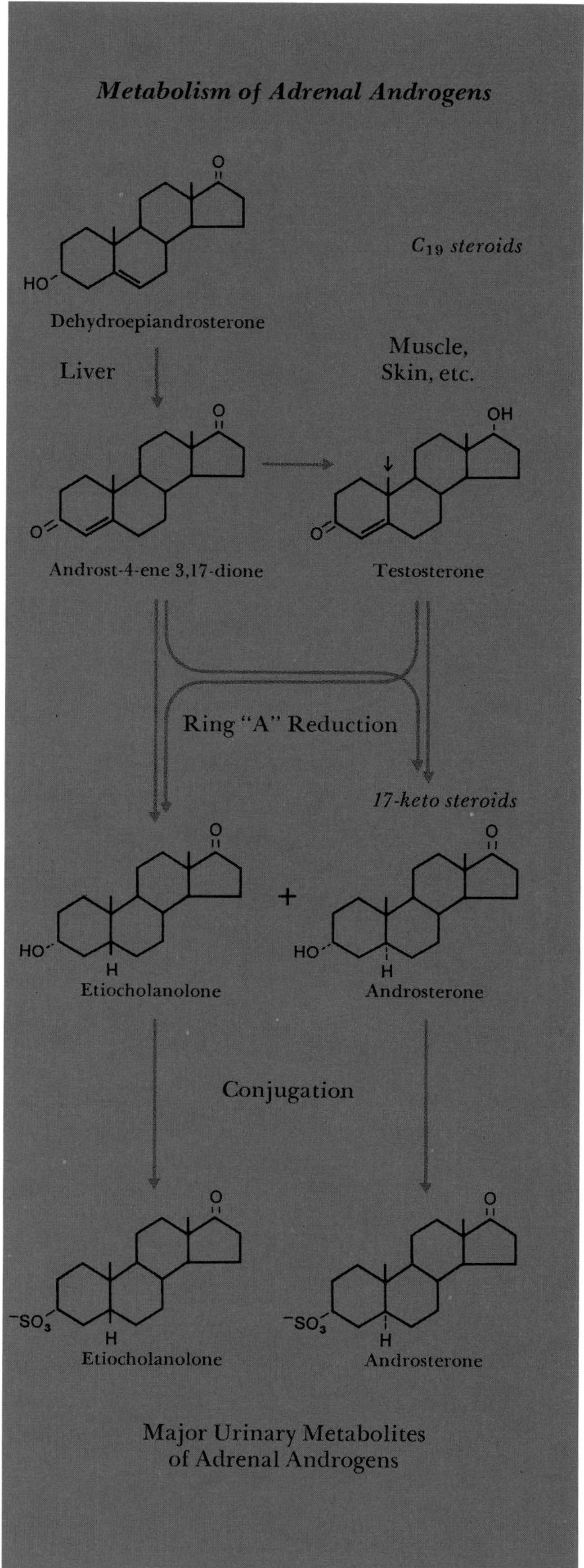

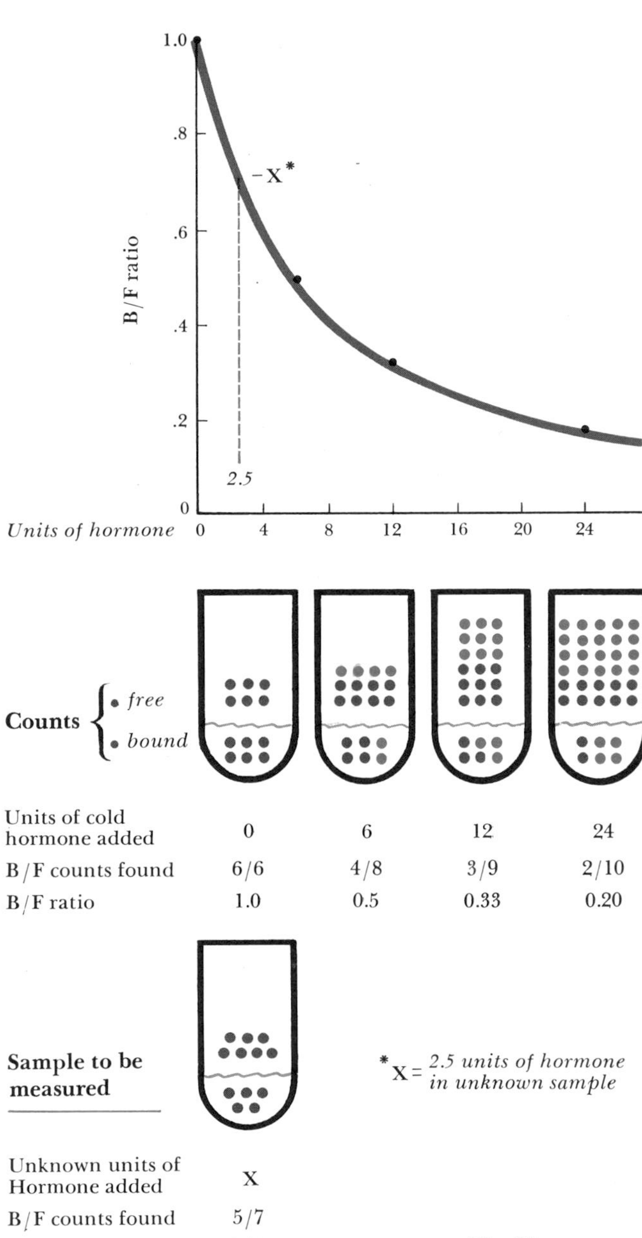

Fig. 33

with the large amount of tetrahydrocortisone and tetrahydrocortisol found in urine compared with serum, makes a fairly accurate and reliable method for assessing the adrenal cortisol secreting function. The normal twenty-four hour excretion rate of 17-OHCS is 2 to 8 mg for the female and 2 to 10 mg for the male. Although tetrahydrocortisol and tetrahydrocortisone do not represent all the urinary metabolites of cortisol, they comprise a fairly constant fraction of cortisol metabolites in the adult. This assay also has the further advantage of measuring the urinary metabolites of 11-deoxycortisol, the compound formed when the metyrapone test is used to investigate adrenal or pituitary function. It should be noted that this method does not measure total 17-hydroxycorticosteroid content for cortolones; cortexolones and pregnanetriol are not measured by this reaction since they have no C-20 ketone group, in spite of containing a 17-hydroxy group. It is conventional, in this country, to use the term urinary 17-OHCS as synonymous with Porter-Silber chromogens and total 17-OHCS as synonymous with the more frequently used 17-ketogenic steroid determination.

17-Ketogenic Steroids: All urinary C_{21} steroids (not C_{19}) containing a 17-OH group can be transformed into a 17-ketosteroid (C_{19}) by a chemical reaction with sodium borohydrate followed by a periodate oxidation (hence the term keto-GENIC). The borohydride reduction reaction destroys the existing 17-ketosteroids in the

Fig. 33 *Principle of the competitive binding method for plasma cortisol. This concept applies to immunoassays and tissue receptor assays utilizing similar radioactive isotope displacement techniques. The assay is based on the principle that at equilibrium, increasing quantities of cold (unlabeled) hormone will displace radioactive tagged cortisol from the binding protein* CBG. *In this instance, an amount of 14C cortisol and* CBG *is added to each tube so that there are equal 14C counts bound to the* CBG *and free in solution (B/F ratio = 1). As increasing amounts of cortisol (unlabeled hormone) are added to each tube, more 14C counts (labeled hormone) are displaced from* CBG *to be free in solution. When the free 14C cortisol counts are adsorbed to charcoal added to the tubes and separated from the* CBG *bound counts by centrifugation, a curve of the 14C counts in the supernatant and centrifugate can be constructed. The cortisol present in a known volume of human plasma is removed by solvent extraction and added to a test tube containing the same amount of* CBG *and 14C cortisol as in the standard curve. Separation and counting of the bound and free hormone allows determination of this ratio. This can then be read on the standard curve to give an accurate estimate of the cortisol content of the sample. Note that the early part of the curve is most sensitive to the addition of cortisol. As the B/F ratio falls, greatly increased amounts of "cold" cortisol must be added to produce even a slight reduction in the B/F ratio. It is therefore necessary to dilute samples so they are read on the earlier more sensitive part of the curve.*

Fig. 34 *Metabolites of adrenal steroids measured by the 17-*KS*, 17-*KGS*, and 17-*OHCS *procedures.*

urine so the 17-ketosteroids newly formed by the periodate oxidation can then be measured by the classic Zimmermann reaction for 17-ketosteroids. In addition to measuring all the usual metabolites of cortisol, this method also measures pregnanetriol, a steroid which may be found in very high concentrations in the urine of patients with the adrenogenital syndrome, and in this instance, 17-ketogenic steroids give a false idea of cortisol production. Some drugs and large amounts of glucose in the urine interfere with this test. *(Fig. 35)* The latter is easily overcome by destroying glucose in the urine sample before beginning the test. The test is simple and less expensive than the Porter-Silber method. It is generally reliable but since the overlap between the normal range of values and some patients with very mild Cushing's syndrome may occur, other maneuvers, subsequently described, may be necessary to make a final diagnosis. Adult males excrete up to 22 milligrams of 17 KGS daily and adult females excrete up to 18 milligrams.

Urinary 17-Ketosteroids: In 1936, not too many years after steroids were known to be present in urine, Dr. Wilhelm Zimmermann in Germany, described a reaction for 17-ketosteroids with sodium metadinitrobenzene that was quickly utilized as a measure of adrenal androgens. For over twenty years the measurement of adrenal steroids as 17-ketosteroids was the only clinically reliable method of estimating adrenocortical function. The test for 17-ketosteroids has now outlived its real usefulness but it still lingers on. The reasons this test should be superseded by newer measures of adrenocortical function are:

a). Traditionally, it was to be a measure of androgenicity by assessing "adrenal androgens" (17-ketosteroids). We now know that all C_{19} steroids secreted by the adrenal are very weakly androgenic in themselves and usually derive their androgenicity by their conversion to testosterone in non-adrenal tissues. Androgenicity, or virilism, is therefore better correlated with plasma testosterone concentration than with urinary 17-ketosteroid excretion and the former is rapidly supplanting urinary 17-ketosteroids as a measure of virilism in the female. Moreover, two-thirds of urinary 17-ketosteroids as measured by this reaction are contributed to by the adrenal and only one-third by the testis as metabolites of testosterone and its precursors. Since testosterone is so much more biologically potent than the adrenal androgens, an increase in plasma testosterone concentration sufficient to produce severe virilism can occur, yet its contribution to the 17-ketosteroid deter-

34

Urinary Metabolites
measured by the
17-OHCS, 17-KS & 17-KGS
Procedures

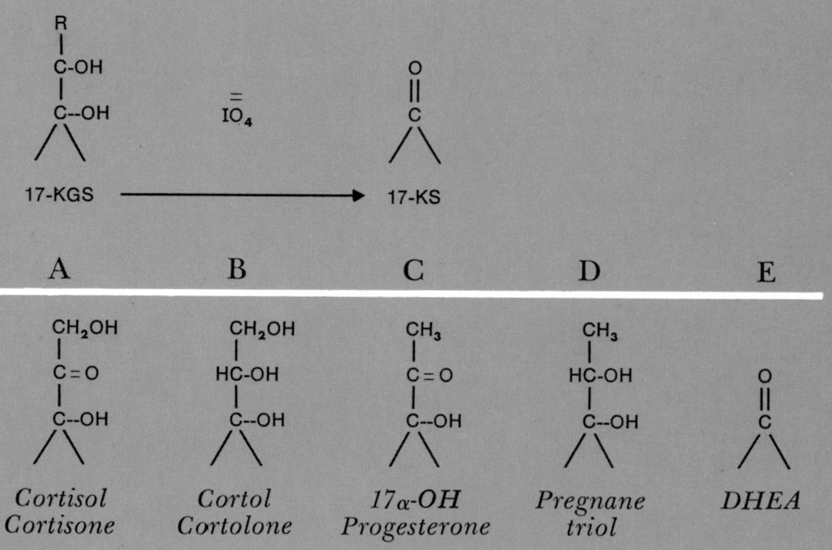

R–C-OH–C--OH (17-KGS) → IO_4 → O=C (17-KS)

	A	B	C	D	E
	CH_2OH / C=O / C--OH	CH_2OH / HC-OH / C--OH	CH_3 / C=O / C--OH	CH_3 / HC-OH / C--OH	O=C
	Cortisol Cortisone	*Cortol Cortolone*	*17α-OH Progesterone*	*Pregnane triol*	*DHEA*
Porter-Silber 17-OHCS	+	–	–	–	–
Zimmermann 17-KS	–	–	–	–	+
$NaBH_4$	B	B	D	D	17-OH
$NaBH_4 + IO_4$	E	E	E	E	–
$NaBH_4 + IO_4$ 17-KGS + Zimmermann	+	+	+	+	–

mination is so small that their measurement may remain well within the normal range.

b). Since such a small proportion of cortisol secreted by the adrenal is metabolized into urinary 17-ketosteroids (approximately 5%) great changes in cortisol secretion can occur without increasing urinary 17-ketosteroid secretion rate outside its rather broad normal range. It is, therefore, a poor measure of adrenocortical function as well as being a very poor measure of virilizing function.

The Zimmermann reaction, however, remains the basis for measuring urinary cortisol metabolites in the 17-ketogenic method since it is simple and reliable. At the moment, measurement of 17 KGS is the best clinical method to assess changes in adrenocortical function. It is possible that with the development of antibodies to cortisol or refinements of the CBG cortisol method, urinary free cortisol measurement might be, in the near future, the best measure of increased adrenocortical function. Normally, free urinary cortisol concentration or excretion rate varies from 50 to 150 ug/day. This represents that small fraction of plasma total cortisol (about 5%) that is filtered through the renal glomerulus and escapes tubular reabsorption. As previously mentioned, CBG is almost maximally saturated at normal plasma cortisol concentrations and a slight increase in the adrenal cortisol secretion rapidly saturates the free CBG sites and inordinately, therefore, increases the proportion of free cortisol present. This is then reflected in a much greater proportionate increase in urinary free cortisol than in the total plasma cortisol measurement, or, indeed, in the urinary metabolites as measured by 17-hydroxycorticosteroids or urinary 17-ketogenic steroids. It also tends to "integrate" all the bursts of plasma cortisol activity known to characterize adrenal secretion in normal subjects and in the majority of patients with Cushing's syndrome. That is, a random plasma cortisol estimation may vary so much within the day that it is difficult to tell whether the total 24-hour secretion rate of cortisol is normal or not. Since all secreted cortisol is eventually metabolized and collected as urine, this tends to be a good measure of the secretion rate of cortisol by the adrenal cortex if there are no abnormalities with urine collection.

Secretion Rates of Adrenocortical Steroids

The actual production rate of cortisol (or aldosterone) can be accurately measured in patients by the use of pure radioactive cortisol (or aldosterone). This measurement depends on the principal of isotope dilution, whereby the radioactive cortisol injected into a patient is diluted by the non-radioactive cortisol secreted by the adrenal cortex. Since the amount of radioactive cortisol given is known, the proportion of radioactive cortisol to non-radioactive cortisol can be found by measurement of non-radioactive plasma cortisol, or by a urinary metabolite of cortisol. This can then be used to calculate the amount of dilution of the radioactive isotope that occurred giving an accurate assessment of the amount of non-radioactive cortisol produced by the adrenal. It is only used when very borderline cases of Cushing's syndrome or Conn's syndrome need to be investigated. Since it involves injection of a radioactive substance into the patient and many chromatographic steps to purify both the radioactive and non-radioactive materials it is not suitable for general clinical use. However, this radioactive material is commercially available and frequently the test may be a crucial diagnostic aid.

35

Drugs *leading to false elevations (↑) or depressions (↓) of chemical determination of urinary 17-KS, 17-KGS, or 17-OHCS*	*17-KS*	*17-KGS*	*17-OHCS*
Hydroxyzine			↑
Chlordiazepoxide HCl	↓		↑
Meprobamate	↑		↑
Nalidixic Acid	↑	↑	→
Oleandomycin	↑		↑
Penicillin	↑	↑	
Phenaglycodol	↑	↑	
Reserpine	↓		↓
Spironolactone	↑		↑
Chlorpromazine	↑		↓
Ethinamate	↑		

Fig. 35 *Drugs leading to false elevation or depression of urinary 17-KS, 17-KGS and 17-OHCS.*

4 Physiology and Pharmacology of Adrenocortical Steroids

Cortisol synthesis and release by the zona fasciculata and zona reticularis of the human adrenal cortex is regulated by the pituitary polypeptide, corticotrophin (adrenocorticotrophin, ACTH). Removal of the pituitary gland in the experimental animal or in man results in functional atrophy and a decrease in weight of the inner zone of the adrenal cortex within a few days. Injections of ACTH increases the secretion rate of cortisol and if prolonged, increases the weight and size of the adrenal cortex two to fourfold. No other control mechanism for cortisol secretion is known. Infusion of cortisol above physiologic concentrations will suppress ACTH release from the pituitary and complete removal of the adrenal leads to a marked increase in the plasma concentration of ACTH. This implies a simple direct negative feedback control for ACTH and cortisol regulation. Yet, in surgical, emotional, or other traumatic stress, ACTH levels in plasma are high despite high concentrations of plasma cortisol which would ordinarily result in non-detectable plasma ACTH measurements. Clearly, a more complex system of regulation requiring close control by the nervous system is operative.

Anatomy: The anterior pituitary gland receives its blood supply, and thereby its control, via a system of portal veins arising in the median eminence of the hypothalamus and terminating in various parts of the anterior pituitary. *(Fig. 36)* Its effluent then drains through veins to the dural sinuses and into the general circulation. The median eminence is a mass of nerve terminals surrounded by perivascular spaces and capillary loops which are called gomotoli bodies. These are the beginning of the portal system flowing to the pituitary and

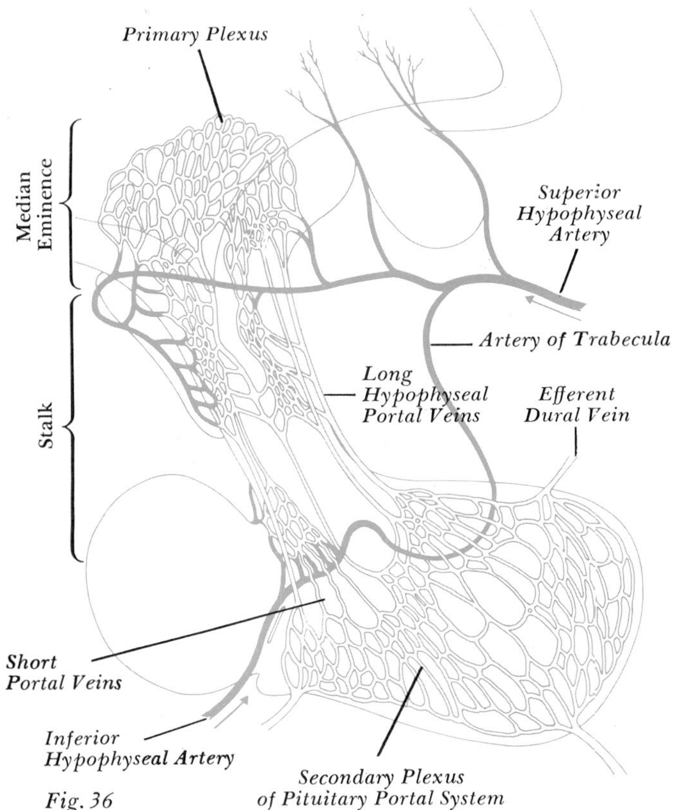

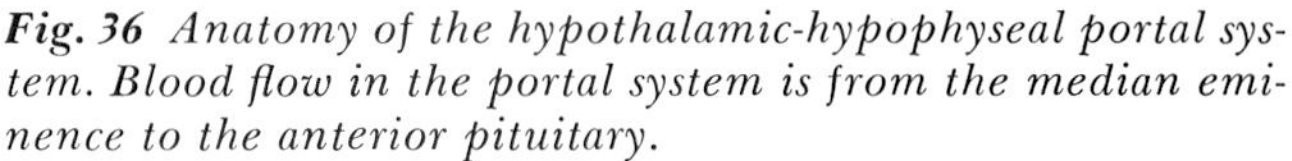
Fig. 36 *Anatomy of the hypothalamic-hypophyseal portal system. Blood flow in the portal system is from the median eminence to the anterior pituitary.*

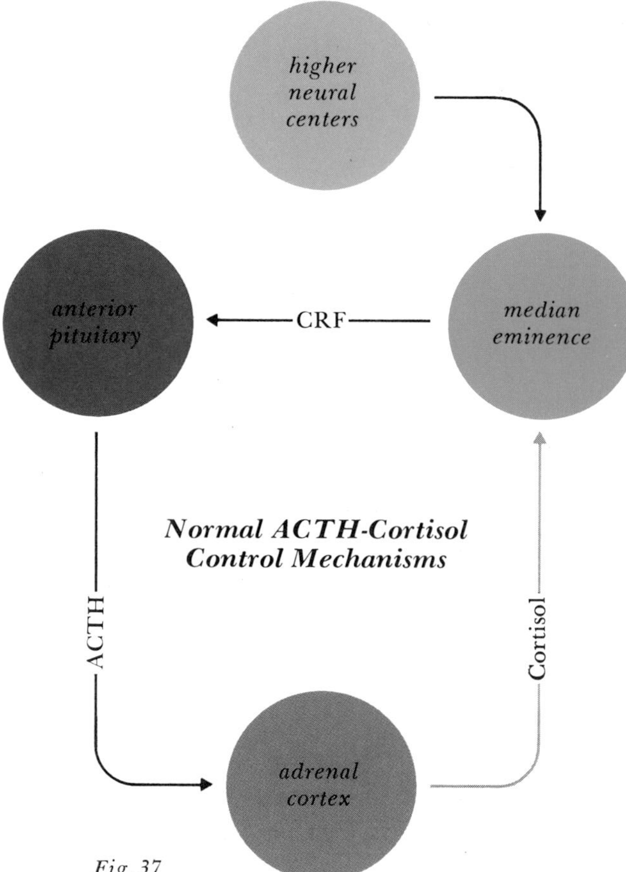

the ending of the arteriolar supply of the median eminence. The median eminence is unlike most of the brain in that there appears to be no "blood-brain" barrier present to impede rapid hormone transfer between nerve cell endings and these capillary loops. In man at least 90% of the blood in the anterior pituitary passes through these structures in the median eminence.

Very few nerves terminate in the anterior pituitary gland, and therefore no direct nervous control is exerted on the pituitary. Control occurs principally via this portal system. ACTH synthesis and release is controlled directly by a small polypeptide, corticotrophin releasing factor (CRF) produced in the median eminence and carried to the basophilic cells of the anterior pituitary by this hypophyseal portal blood. CRF is in reality a central nervous system hormone connecting the complex neurophysiologic reactions of "stress" via the anterior pituitary to the adrenal cortex.

Control

In the resting state ACTH and cortisol bear a reciprocal control relationship to one another. ACTH release produces a rise in plasma cortisol which in turn acts on receptors in the median eminence to decrease CRF secretion and thus reduce ACTH release. *(Fig. 37)* As the effective level of hydrocortisone falls off in some as yet unknown receptor site within the median eminence or hypothalamus, CRF secretion increases and then the cycle is complete. This simple servomechanism can be overridden by other stimuli originating in other centers of the CNS. This occurs during "stress". Complex CNS responses stimulate CRF secretion even in the presence of high circulating plasma concentrations of cortisol. This is a complex response and probably more than a simple readjustment of the "set-point" to the higher level of tissue receptor cortisol, for even massive doses of glucocorticoid will not suppress ACTH release in severe acute stress. Such severe stress can increase the adrenal secretion of steroids from five to tenfold.

Diurnal (Circadian) Cortisol Secretion

It has been known for many years that plasma cortisol concentration is much higher in the early morning than through the afternoon and evening. This diurnal or circadian rhythm was difficult to reconcile with a negative feedback control without postulating that central nervous system activity altered the feedback re-

Fig. 37 *Control of cortisol secretion by* ACTH *is modulated by a negative feed-back system on the hypothalamic receptors and by higher neural centers.*

Fig. 38 *The diurnal curve of plasma cortisol is actually composed of irregular bursts of* ACTH *and cortisol secretion. The "bursts" occur more frequently in the early morning and give rise to the "circadian-rhythm" of cortisol shown by the smooth curve.*

ceptor set in a daily rhythmical manner. Recent evidence has shown that, in man, the smooth rhythm of cortisol concentration depicted is not entirely true but that plasma cortisol is secreted in "bursts" with high peaks and low valleys and that ACTH and cortisol secretion are not continuous but occur in sporadic bursts and that the diurnal pattern seen stems from the fact that most of the ACTH-cortisol bursts occur in the early morning, peaking out between 4 a.m. and 8 a.m. in the average normal subject. *(Fig. 38)* This mechanism is of concern for it is possible that the cause of Cushing's syndrome in many patients lies in a disturbance of this mechanism and that careful study of "bursting rhythms" may not only be a clue to the genesis of Cushing's syndrome but may be valuable in its diagnosis.

Biological Effects

The major glucocorticoid produced by the adrenal cortex of man, cortisol, has a mild mineralocorticoid effect. The major mineralocorticoid, aldosterone, has a mild glucocorticoid effect. Both steroids exert their action on cellular metabolism by entering the cell and stimulating or controlling new protein synthesis. They also appear directly or indirectly to inhibit or alter membrane integrity and membrane transport systems. The new proteins formed are usually enzymes. This effect is particularly evident in the liver. In cells there appear to be specific binding proteins for steroids, both in the nucleus and on the ribosomes of the endoplasmic reticulum. Several theories as to their mode of promoting both messenger RNA and ribosomal protein synthesis have been proposed but no single concept has yet been proven that is generally acceptable to all investigators.

In certain tissues other than liver, such as muscle, bone and lymphoid tissue, high concentrations of glucocorticoids are catabolic and appear to inhibit protein synthesis, possibly by interfering with RNA synthesis leading to an unopposed breakdown of protein and thereby to amino acid release. Cortisol also directly inhibits the uptake and metabolism of glucose in skin and adipose tissue. In contrast to these inhibitory effects, cortisol is anabolic in the liver.

Here cortisol increases the transport of amino acids into the liver cell. By inducing RNA synthesis it increases the production of a number of enzymes which are concerned with the conversion of the carbon skeleton of the amino acids to glucose and glycogen. This leads directly to deposition of glycogen as a consequence of this increased gluconeogenesis. This effect is well accepted and it is from this action that the term glucocorticoid first arose. The overall effect of cortisol on energy metabolism of the organism is to supplant and conserve the energy derived from circulating glucose. This is accomplished by inhibiting glucose utilization in peripheral tissues; by mediating a flow of amino acids to the liver for new glucose synthesis; by promoting a shift in muscle tissue energy sources from glucose to fatty acid metabolism and by mobilizing fatty acids from adipose tissue. The initial action of cortisol to inhibit glycolysis in peripheral tissue is probably aided by a superimposed inhibition of key glycolytic enzymes by the increased circulating free fatty acids.

In all these actions there is a delay of two to four hours before the steroid effect is manifest, clearly compatible with the induction of new protein and enzyme synthesis by an action on the gene of the cell. Many of these described effects have been discovered by *in vitro* studies or by the administration of cortisol or other glucocorticoids to adrenalectomized animals, or by giving doses of cortisol much greater than those normally present, to animals or man. Despite years of investigation there is a great uncertainty as to how and what cortisol really does at normal tissue concentrations. There is wide acceptance of the concept of Engel, suggesting that cortisol exerts a "permissive" action on metabolic and enzyme function throughout cellular tissue, thus permitting a variety of other hormones and agents to exert their effect. In certain instances these permissive effects are clearly an induction of enzyme synthesis (adipose lipase, liver gluconeogenic enzymes) which then are activated by other hormones, e.g., glucagon.

38

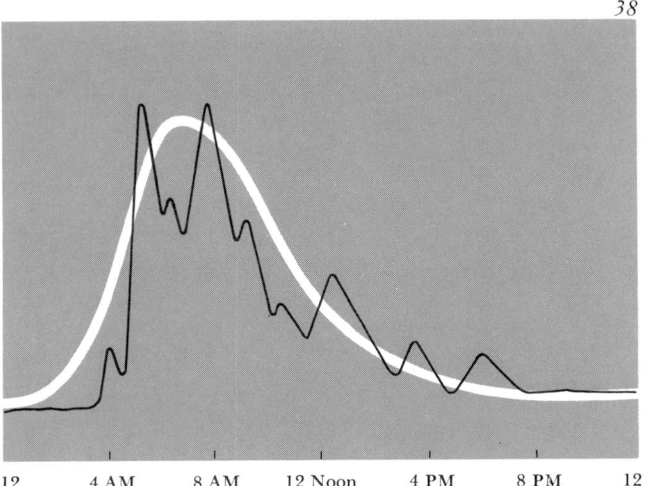

Pharmacology

When used to treat hypoadrenalism, cortisol and mineralocorticoid are used in physiologic replacement doses. Since Addison's Disease is very rare, the average physician does not often use steroids for this purpose.

Yet, steroids are one of the most frequently prescribed drugs in this country. This is because when used in pharmacologic doses, glucocorticoids possess remarkable anti-inflammatory effects. However, to gain this beneficial action the side effects may be of a severity that the benefits are not worthwhile. In simple terms, the cure may be worse than the disease.

Beneficial Effects of Pharmacologic Doses of Adrenocortical Steroids

Anti-inflammatory effects: The dramatic demonstration of the beneficial action of cortisone in rheumatoid arthritis by Hench in 1948 initiated the pharmacologic use of steroids. Since then it has been shown that this action is possessed only by pure glucocorticoid hormones and not by pure mineralocorticoid hormones. Vascular permeability is decreased, capillary resistance is increased and the vasoconstrictive effect of norepinephrine is potentiated. This latter effect on capillaries may be an immediate action occurring within minutes and can be dramatically demonstrated by dropping steroid containing solution directly on living rabbit omentum when viewed with a dissecting microscope. It is possible glucocorticoids suppress the release or action of histamine on surrounding tissues. The migration of inflammatory cells from capillaries is depressed. These effects reduce inflammatory tissue swelling by lessening edema fluid formation and prevent swelling and distortion of cells by maintaining cell wall integrity to water. In addition to this effect on water migration, direct injury to the cell wall by toxins and enzymes may be lessened by a cell wall stabilizing effect of glucocorticoids.

Lymphoid tissue involution: Glucocorticoids produce a striking suppression of lymphoid tissue activity and formation. This effect is manifest in blood as lymphopenia and this action is the basis for steroid treatment of acute and chronic lymphocytic leukemia. Eosinophil counts are decreased by glucocorticoids so consistently that a low eosinophil count was at one time used as an indicator of excess cortisol activity in man. Neutrophilic polymorphonucleocytes are markedly increased by cortisol administration. This is more likely due to decreased destruction and egress of mature leucocytes from the capillaries, than to suppressed bone marrow formation.

Anti-allergy effects: The obvious lymphocytolytic effect of glucocorticoids has been used to suppress immune response in those diseased states related to hyperimmunity. Because of this, in very recent years, glucocorticoids have played a vital role in human organ transplantation operations by preventing or ameliorating the post-transplant response related to organ rejection by the host.

The anti-allergic action of glucocorticoids seems primarily mediated through a suppression of the inflammatory response that results from antigen-antibody induced injury. Steroids do not interfere with antigen-antibody interaction and in man, at least in the usual doses used for therapy, do not significantly suppress antibody formation. If the therapeutic dose is very high and maintained for long periods of time new antibody formation is, however, depressed, probably through lymphocytolysis and suppressed gamma globulin formation. This effect begins after the first week of high dose therapy and the long delay for the action to occur must be recognized when managing certain autoimmune diseases, or when anticipated transplant reactions, such as to kidney transplants, are being managed. In tissues, antigen-antibody interaction leads to histamine release with a resultant inflammatory response. Glucocorticoids must be directly present in high concentration at this site to prevent or lessen this response. Steroids probably do not suppress histamine release but only oppose its tissue effects. If the tissue is poorly accessible to plasma-borne steroids, extremely high doses must be given to produce acceptable concentrations of steroid at the actual site of the inflammation.

Lysosomal stabilization effects: Recently, attention has been drawn to the role that lysosomes may play in disease. Lysosomes are small sacs located within the cytoplasm of cells. They contain a variety of potentially destructive hydrolytic enzymes which, however, are prevented from destroying the intracellular content of the cell by the sac membrane. A number of factors (ischemia, endotoxins, x-rays, streptolycin) may disrupt these sacs, releasing their contents and producing severe cellular injury. Glucocorticoids apparently stabilize the membranes, prevent diffusion of the enzymes into the cell and thereby prevent digestion of the cell contents. This action decreases the spread of inflammation from this cell injury as it migrates through enzyme dispersal from cell to cell. The mechanism of glucocorticoid stabilization of the lysosomal membrane is unknown. This action may also affect membranes of other intracellular organelles. This is not a unique effect of glucocorticoids for other agents are also known to stabilize lysosomal membranes.

Anti-stress effects: Largely through the efforts of Hans Selye beginning in the late 1930's the concept arose that innumerable noxious stimuli on the body were followed by a host of similar defense mechanisms, prominent among which was adrenocortical steroid discharge. The term "stress" gradually became accepted as the blanket term for those noxious stimuli which led to the death of adrenalectomized animals. In turn, such animals were protected from the stress if adrenocortical extracts were given prior to the stress. In a curious manner this concept influenced research on steroids at a time when most medical research activities were in abeyance, i.e., World War II. In a fascinating tale related by Kendall, the discoverer of cortisone, rumors were spread in Allied war circles that Luftwaffe pilots were receiving injections of adrenocortical extracts that enabled them to withstand the stress of low oxygen-high altitude flying and converted them to "supermen." This led to intensified efforts to isolate the potent principle of adrenocortical extracts and to study their physiologic effects in man on this side of the Atlantic. Although the rumor and the effects of adrenocortical extract proved untrue, it eventually led to the synthesis of cortisone and its utilization in rheumatoid arthritis by Hench. Since then a great deal of research on this stress phenomenon has accumulated but a fundamental understanding of the role played by adrenocortical steroids in body defenses is lacking.

When the human undergoes stress such as a surgical operation, a major illness or a severe automobile accident, plasma ACTH and cortisol concentration increase rapidly and remain high for a considerable time, i.e., stress has overcome the "negative feedback" control mechanism to allow the body to better withstand the stress. *(Fig. 39)* In the adrenalectomized patient, if steroids are not given during this stress, the patient will die in acute vascular collapse. This adrenal response is "physiologic" since the adrenocortical response to stress has been found to be limited. Under maximal stress the normal human adrenal glands can produce only 200 to 300 mg of cortisol per day. The concept arose that many stresses might be more than physiologic and for adequate bodily defense might require larger amounts of steroid than the maximally stimulated adrenal cortex could produce. This is probably true. Pharmacologic doses (1 to 3 grams of cortisol) seem to aid in the treatment of such overwhelming diseases as gram negative septicemia and septic shock.

The major body response to overwhelming stress is

Fig. 39 *ACTH and cortisol increase with the stress of surgical operation. Both usually return to normal within 24 hours following the procedure. Patients with severe burns may show increased concentrations for several days.*

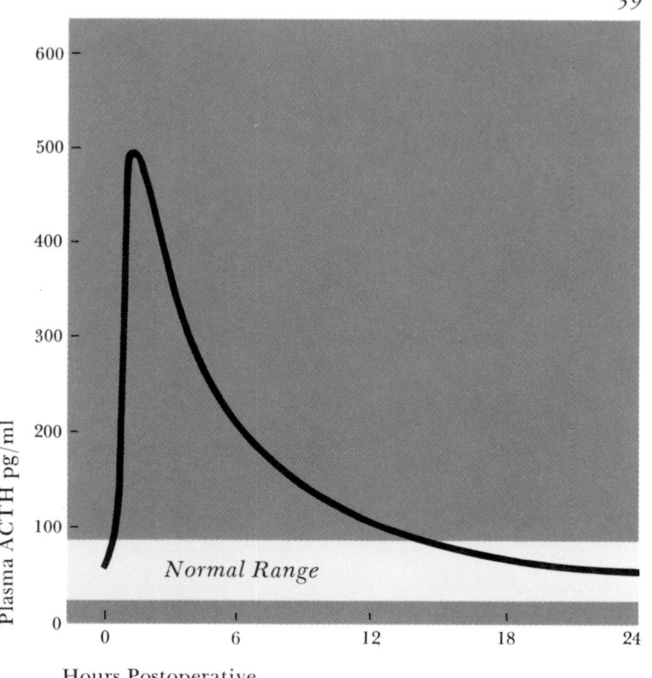

vascular collapse. How adrenocortical steroids help restore this reaction to normal is controversial. There is evidence that glucocorticoids enhance the vasoconstrictive action of norepinephrine but that they prevent the excessive vasoconstriction which leads to tissue ischema by directly acting on vascular smooth muscle and that they directly stimulate the myocardium. These actions are disputed and many believe metabolic effects are more important, i.e., evidence suggests steroids act in stress by: 1. preventing lactate accumulation; 2. suppressing histamine release; 3. inducing key oxidative enzyme formation; 4. directly antagonizing toxins and kinins; 5. directly stabilizing lysosomal membranes.

The role of the adrenocortical response to stress is unclear, but the following points should be emphasized: 1. An increase in plasma cortisol is essential for man to withstand severe stress; 2. Glucocorticoids alone have this affect; 3. Supraphysiologic "stress" may require a supraphysiologic dose of glucocorticoids to maintain life processes.

Adverse Effects

Except for the protective effect of physiologic doses of cortisol in adrenal insufficiency, the previously enumerated beneficial effects of steroids are generally found only when corticosteroid secretion rates are two to three times normal, i.e., 40 to 60 mg per day or higher, or in the pharmacologic range, i.e., greater than 200 to 300 mg per day. When equivalent doses of cortisol are given as a synthetic cortisol-like steroid, these beneficial actions are usually accompanied by, or produce adverse effects which seriously limit their use as drugs. These adverse effects may begin to appear at any dosage above normal resting secretion rates.

Since cortisone and cortisol have a slight mineralocorticoid action in pharmacologic doses, they may produce adverse effects on water and electrolyte metabolism. The adverse effects of cortisol may therefore be grouped as glucocorticoid and mineralocorticoid. The second group can be largely ignored because one of the major therapeutic advances in steroid treatment of disease has been the synthesis of steroids almost completely devoid of mineralocorticoid action, while retaining full or enhanced glucocorticoid effect. There has been no steroid produced which will completely separate one glucocorticoid effect from another. Therefore, the potential side effects of the drug must be considered whenever beneficial effects are required.

Glucocorticoid Side Effects

In general the toxic effects of glucocorticoids are manifest as excessive catabolism of tissues other than the liver. Those patients with "pure" Cushing's syndrome who secrete only cortisol present these manifestations.

Diabetes—The anti-insulin-like effects of cortisol lead to an abnormal glucose tolerance test or to mild diabetes mellitus in about one quarter to one third of patients on chronic treatment with glucocorticoid.

Muscle weakness—The protein catabolic effect of glucocorticoids leads to muscle weakness and in severe cases to muscle atrophy.

Skin disorders—Easy bruisability and reddish striae develop because of thinning of the skin. Interference with protein synthesis and the often attendant rapidly increasing obesity seen around the region of the hips, thighs and shoulders seem to produce this. Additionally, wound repair is delayed.

Obesity—The overall affect of glucocorticoids on fat is to induce a redistribution and slight increase in central body fat. Free fatty acids are mobilized by cortisol infusions. In the long term, central obesity with a moon face and reddened plethoric cheeks are characteristic of this overall effect.

Peptic ulcer—Although peptic ulcer is not common in Cushing's syndrome, the oral administration of glucocorticoids seems to be associated with a slight increase in peptic ulcerogenesis. If the ulcers bleed, serious consequences of steroid overdosage can rapidly ensue.

Osteoporosis—One of the most serious and unfortunately irreversible effects of glucocorticoid overdosage is loss of bone substance.

Growth suppression—In children, another irreversible effect of excessive steroid dosage is failure of longitudinal bone growth. Thus, in long term treatment of childhood allergic illness with steroids, an exceptionally hazardous side effect is encountered.

Cataract—Central cataract formation, particularly in the young, is a serious and irreversible effect.

Virilism—Though often seen as manifest acne and hirsutism in Cushing's syndrome, true hirsutism is unknown in pure glucocorticoid overdosage. An increase in lanugo type hair occurs but the dark terminal hairs characteristic of hirsutism and virilism as seen in Cushing's syndrome is absent. In Cushing's syndrome, however, this is due to the metabolism of adrenal androgens to testosterone.

Infection—In the presence of increased cortisol, the ability of the host defense mechanism to overcome bacterial invasion may be inhibited. Serious and rapid spread of an established infection may occur if it is not simultaneously treated with antibiotics and other necessary measures.

Menses—Treatment with excessive glucocorticoids is often attended by irregular or absent menstruation. The mechanism for this is not known. In small doses, steroids have been used to regularize the irregular menses seen in the Stein-Leventhal syndrome.

Mental effects—Steroids have unpredictable and profound effects on the psyche. This can be a result of excessive steroid dosage and is also seen when steroid replacement therapy in Addison's Disease is insufficient. Large doses of steroids may lead to insomnia. In a considerable number of patients there is initial euphoria and in long term therapy a number of psychotic manifestations may occur. A frequent problem is depression. Withdrawal of the steroids does not necessarily lead to remission of the mental side effects.

ACTH suppression and adrenal atrophy—Within a beginning week of glucocorticoid treatment in man, adrenocortical atrophy begins because of the continuous suppression of ACTH release from the pituitary. This is due to inhibition of CRF release from the median eminence. This effect may be seen at any dose greater than the equivalent of the normal daily secretion of cortisol, i.e., 30 mg/day. All synthetic glucocorticoids possess this ACTH suppressant effect in direct proportion to their glucocorticoid potency. Cortisol, if given as a single oral dose of 30 mg is rapidly absorbed and will suppress ACTH within thirty minutes. The half-life of cortisol is short and measurably elevated levels in plasma will have disappeared in six to eight hours. The suppressant effect lasts somewhat longer and ACTH will only begin to be secreted twelve to sixteen hours later. If no further cortisol is taken, ACTH will rise and lead to secretion of cortisol from the adrenals. Adrenal atrophy is not likely to occur under these circumstances with daily medication. However, it has been shown that this dose, if slowly infused or released over twenty-four hours, will keep ACTH continuously suppressed. Suppression of the adrenal cortex is therefore more duration dependent than dose dependent. A small dose continuously absorbed will produce much more severe suppression than a large dose intermittently given. However, a single large dose will produce longer suppression than a small dose simply because its disappearance from plasma is prolonged. In chronic treatment, as long as possible spacing between doses capable

40

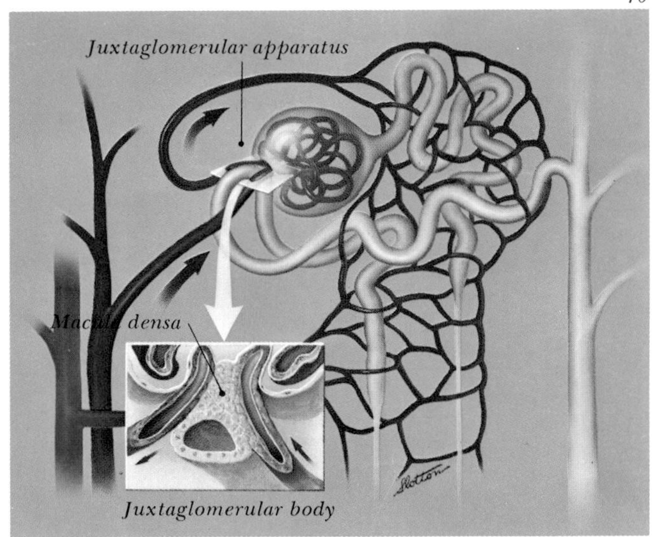

of controlling the condition requiring steroid therapy should be used. This has led to therapy with large doses of steroids every other day, so-called "alternate-day" therapy.

Mineralocorticoid Side Effects

Sodium retention: In the normal subject sodium and water retention with a weight gain of two to four kilograms occurs in the first two to three days of excess cortisol administration. Weight equilibrium is quickly achieved and is followed by a leveling off and escape from the effect, so that sodium intake equals urinary output. However, if it is given to a patient with cardiac failure, escape does not occur; peripheral and pulmonary edema result.

Potassium loss: Sodium-potassium exchange leads to a total body potassium loss with attendant alkalosis and bicarbonate retention. Muscle cramps and muscle weakness occur if the potassium loss is severe.

Hypertension: Long-term treatment with cortisol leads to diastolic hypertension brought about by an unknown mechanism.

These effects are not usually seen with pure synthetic glucocorticoids that are practically devoid of mineralocorticoid effects, i.e., prednisolone and its analogues.

Aldosterone

Aldosterone synthesis and release by the zona glomerulosa is regulated by several factors, the relative importance of which is not yet completely settled. These are: renin-angiotensin, sodium, potassium, ACTH, and unknown factors.

The renin-angiotensin system is the prime regulator of aldosterone secretion and release. Since aldosterone is concerned with body fluid volume regulation, it is understandable that body fluid volume regulates aldosterone release. This is a form of negative feedback control. Renin is secreted in response to extra-renal, intravascular fluid volume depletion, and to intra-renal signals from the macula densa by the specialized myoepithelial cells of the juxtaglomerular apparatus. These cells "cuff" the afferent arterioles of each glomerulus and appear to monitor intrarenal arteriolar pressure by stretch perception. *(Fig. 40)* Renin then released within the renal circulation leads to increased angiotensin production in the circulation which then acts on the adrenal glomerulosa to secrete aldosterone. *(Fig. 41)*

Fig. 40 *The juxtaglomerular apparatus consists of a juxtaglomerular body and the macula densa. It is situated at the junction of the afferent arteriole and the distal tubule. The macula densa is believed to monitor sodium content of the distal tubule, and thus modulate the activity of the juxtaglomerular body.*

Fig. 41 *Schema of aldosterone control through the renin angiotensin system.*

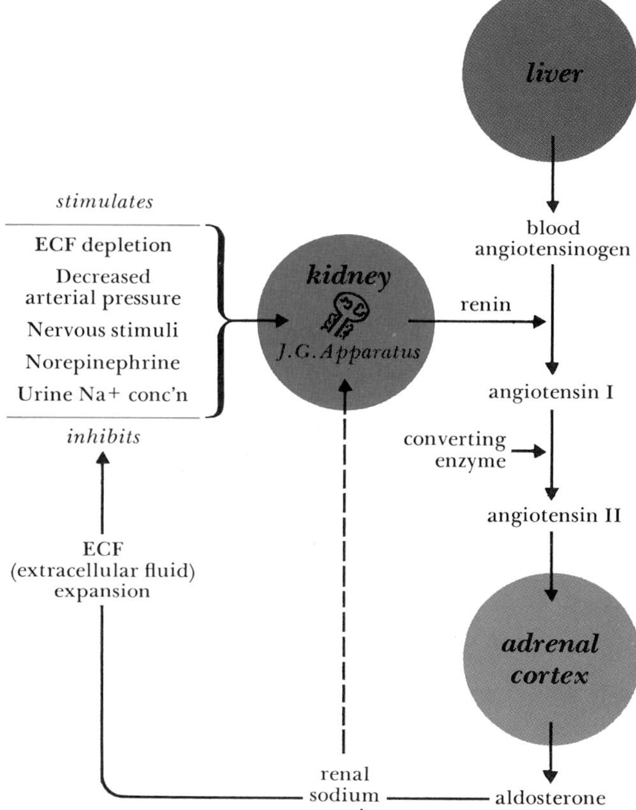

Fig. 41

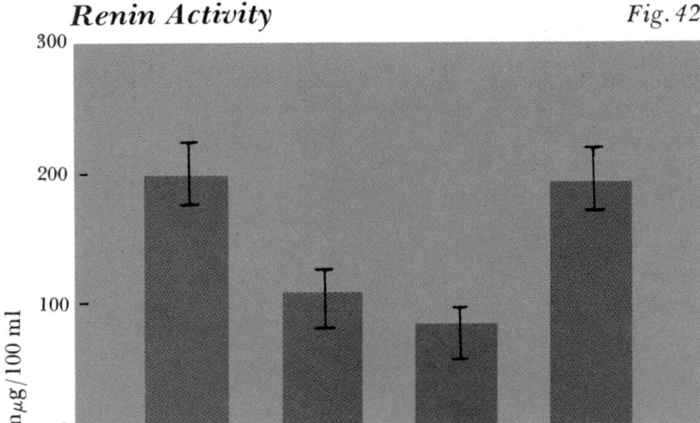

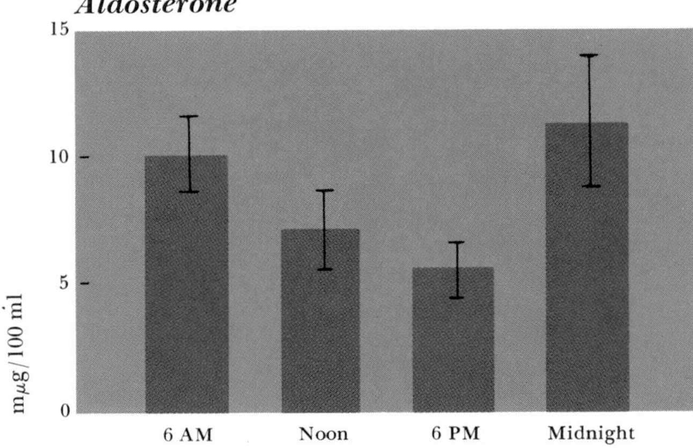

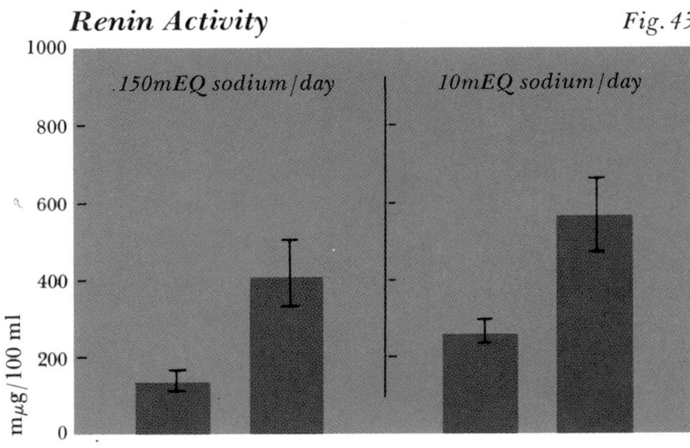

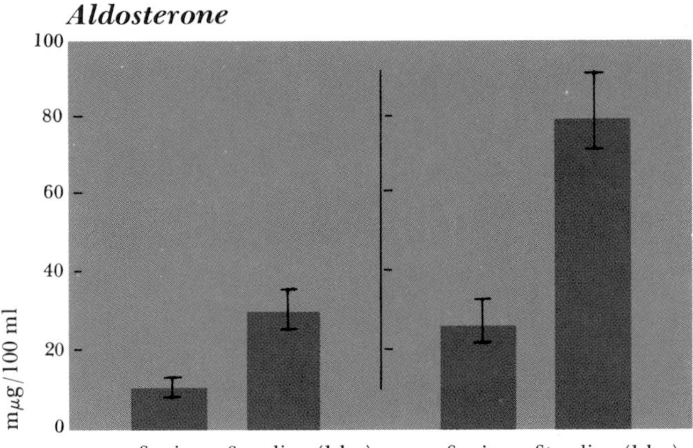

Thus an acute blood loss due to hemorrhage would be perceived by the juxtaglomerular apparatus as a decreased stretch (pressure and/or blood flow), which would lead to slow volume restoration by causing through aldosterone, sodium induced water retention until the "stretch" tension was restored to normal. Conversely, salt overload would be perceived as increased stretch and lead to less sodium retention through decreased aldosterone production.

There is evidence that intrarenal mechanisms sense the sodium concentration in the fluid in the distal tubules via the macula densa. How this is effected is uncertain, but the close apposition of these cells in the distal tubular epithelium with the juxtaglomerular apparatus suggests some direct intercellular control. For example, if a large sodium load is presented to the distal tubule, the macula densa would sense this, cause the juxtaglomerular apparatus to release renin and the resultant aldosterone increase would decrease the sodium loss. This mechanism is evidently a modifier of juxtaglomerular control through the renin angiotensin system. Its precise importance is not yet known.

Sodium—Any of the many factors which affect blood volume will alter the renin-angiotensin system to regain or maintain homeostasis. In the normal human, sodium ion regulation is a prime determinant of body fluid volumes. Almost all sodium ingested is absorbed and then excreted by the kidneys. Exquisite balancing of sodium ion intake versus sodium ion output by the kidney maintains normal body fluid compartments. Sodium ion does not appear to directly influence adrenal secretion of aldosterone except via volume receptors through the renin-angiotensin system or the macula densa.

Potassium—In the experimental animal and in renoprival man there is evidence to suggest that potassium, unlike sodium, directly affects adrenal glomerulosa release of aldosterone. Since aldosterone promotes renal potassium loss it is not surprising that high cellular potassium directly stimulates aldosterone release. It is not yet known whether this is of physiologic significance but in clinical practice it is well known that the low serum potassium concentrations found in some patients with aldosterone producing tumors may be associated with a surprisingly low aldosterone excretion rate. Restoration of body potassium stores by oral potassium supplements often raises the aldosterone excretion rate to

Fig. 42 *Renin and aldosterone in man have a cyclical variation similar to cortisol. This pattern may be largely modulated through* ACTH *secretion.*

Fig. 43 *Effect of salt restriction and assumption of the upright posture on renin and aldosterone concentration.*

Fig. 44 *Molecular road map of the mechanism by which aldosterone is thought to control sodium re-absorption in the distal renal tubule.*

greater than normal. The elevated aldosterone excretion rate presupposed to exist before potassium depletion became evident, is thus restored. A rule of thumb to follow is "if a patient with decreased potassium is suspected of having primary aldosteronism, normal aldosterone excretion rates should not be used to rule out the presence of a tumor until body potassium has been restored to normal".

ACTH—In hypophysectomized man, aldosterone excretion continues, but at a reduced rate, and the response of aldosterone to sodium deprivation is somewhat blunted. Conversely, ACTH infusions to hypophysectomized man result in a slight increase in aldosterone secretion. ACTH seems to be required to keep the aldosterone synthesizing machinery normal but it does not otherwise appear to play an important role in the regulation of body fluids through aldosterone.

44

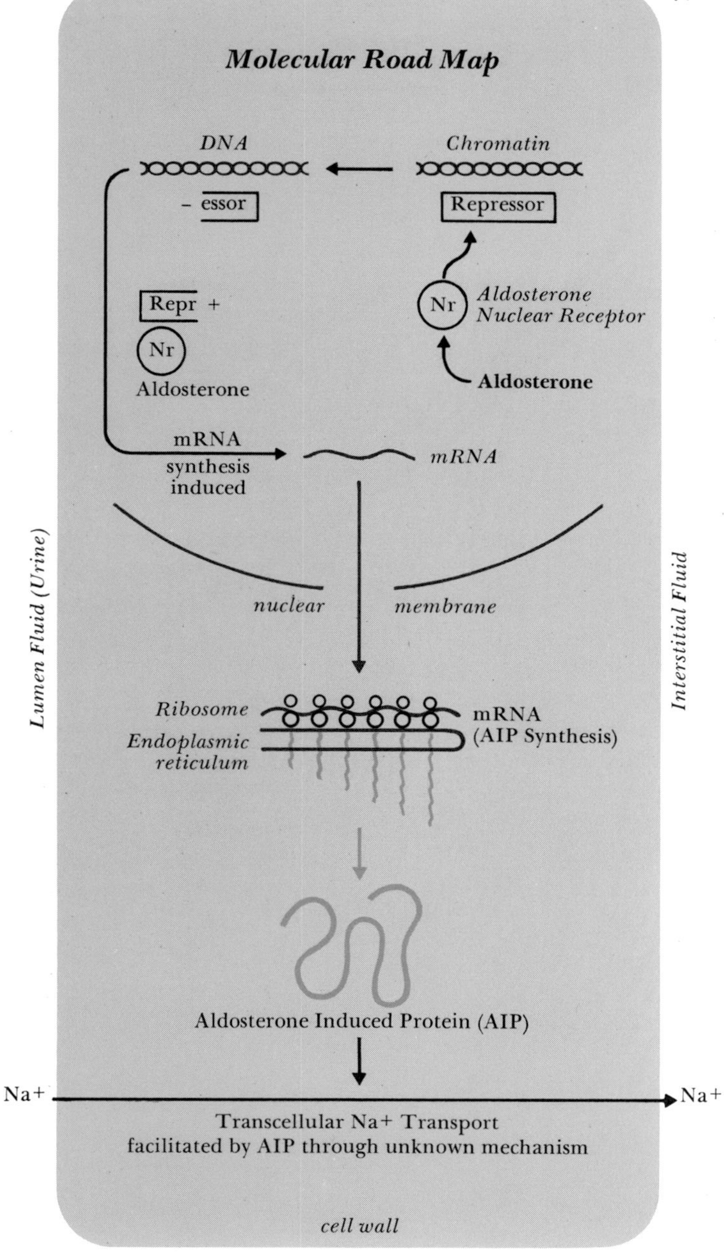

Renal Tubular Epithelium

Control of aldosterone secretion has been studied for over fifteen years. Many experiments in man and animals cannot be accounted for by any of the foregoing control mechanisms, and it is probable that other unknown factors are involved in aldosterone control and body fluid homeostasis.

It is amazing how well the patient with treated Addison's disease without a responsive glucocorticoid or aldosterone secreting mechanism maintains body fluid compartments in a normal state. In fact, almost all patients with Addison's disease maintain perfect health on a daily fixed intake of glucocorticoid and mineralocorticoid despite wide variations in salt and water intake. This leads to the inescapable conclusion that regardless of the proposed mechanism of aldosterone control, changes in aldosterone concentration are relatively unimportant in usual sodium and fluid homeostatic regulation. It appears to be "permissive." If enough is available, other far more important regulators of salt and water metabolism apparently keep body fluids and electrolytes in balance. As yet, these regulators are not defined.

However, when aldosterone secretion mechanisms become disordered and result in excess aldosterone secretion or when an autonomous aldosterone secreting adrenal tumor forms, edema or hypertension results in life-threatening disease. It is in this realm that a knowledge of aldosterone pathophysiology is important to the physician.

Variations of Plasma Aldosterone Concentrations

Circadian variation of plasma aldosterone concentration is present but less obvious than for plasma cortisol *(Fig. 42)*; however, marked postural changes in plasma renin and aldosterone occur, and if not properly understood, they can lead to erroneous interpretations of plasma aldosterone measurements. *(Fig. 43)* An upright standing position leads to a shift in fluid to the lower extremities away from the central volume receptors to the kidney. This leads to elevated renin and aldosterone plasma concentration, which returns to a basal level with horizontal resting. Alterations in this plasma concentration relationship to posture occur in diseased states and are sought for by the clinician as a sign of disorder of the system.

Mineralocorticoid Action

Aldosterone stimulates active sodium reabsorption and sodium-potassium transport across the membranes of many epithelial tissues which are specialized for this function, such as intestinal mucosa, salivary glands, sweat glands and of course, the kidneys. The major site of action is the distal tubule of the renal nephron where it facilitates the reabsorption of sodium and the secretion of potassium. There is some dispute as to whether a similar effect on sodium reabsorption also occurs in the proximal tubule. How aldosterone mediates this action is unknown. It is probable that aldosterone enters the tubular epithelial cell where it binds with specific receptors and induces the synthesis of specific RNA. This new RNA then directs the synthesis of a specific protein which enhances trans-cellular transport of sodium by acting on the rate-limiting step in the sodium transport system. *(Fig. 44)* There are several theories as to how this may be accomplished, but as yet no single mechanism seems to satisfy all observations. We must await further research before assigning more specific sites of action for this Aldosterone Induced Protein. In keeping with this mechanism is the observation that following infusion of aldosterone directly into an isolated kidney, twenty to thirty minutes minimum time elapses before potassium excretion or sodium retention occurs.

In excess, the pharmacologic or pathologic effects of mineralocorticoids are more obvious. *(Fig. 45)* Renal sodium retention is sharply increased when aldosterone injections are given to normal human beings. Water retention occurs and body weight rises 2 to 4 kilograms. However, before edema becomes evident, an "escape" from this sodium retaining effect of the mineralocorticoid occurs and renal sodium and water losses return to approximately equal intake. This escape phenomenon is not present in diseased states such as congestive heart failure, nephrosis and ascites so that the patients continue to gain fluid and retain salt with resultant massive edema. At the same time, potassium excretion is increased. Little or no escape occurs from this latter effect and eventually the subject may become potassium depleted.This leads to alkalosis, bicarbonate retention and muscle weakness.

The "escape" is presumably due to inhibition of proximal tubular sodium resorption by an elusive "third factor," at one time thought to be a "salt wasting" adrenal hormone. (Factor 1 is filtration rate, factor 2 is aldosterone.) In congestive heart failure there is presumed inhibition of third factor release.

The excess retention of sodium in man is related to the development of diastolic hypertension. However, it is exceedingly difficult to demonstrate this in normal man by injections of aldosterone for as long as one month. Such hypertension is, however, seen in patients with Addison's disease overtreated with a synthetic mineralocorticoid for several months. Although hypertension in association with an aldosterone secreting tumor of the adrenal gland is usual, the more common secondary causes of excessive aldosterone associated with edematous states rarely lead to hypertension. It is unknown why patients with primary hyperaldosteronism have hypertension, and why those with secondary hyperaldosteronism do not.

Aldosterone Antagonists

The demonstration that a steroid, progesterone, produced a sodium diuresis in the normal animal, led to the recognition that this action was only observed in the presence of adrenal salt retaining hormones. No such effect occurred in the adrenalectomized animal unless a mineralocorticoid was present. This suggested the action of aldosterone was antagonized at the renal tubule by progesterone. Since then several synthetic steroid analogues have been produced for use as diuretics. *(Fig. 46)* These substances, called spironolactones, have proven useful in the diagnosis and pre-operative management of patients with primary aldosteronism. They restore serum potassium to normal and often reduce the hypertension of primary aldosteronism to normal levels. They appear to act as competitive inhibitors of aldosterone by blocking the specific binding sites of aldosterone on nuclear proteins.

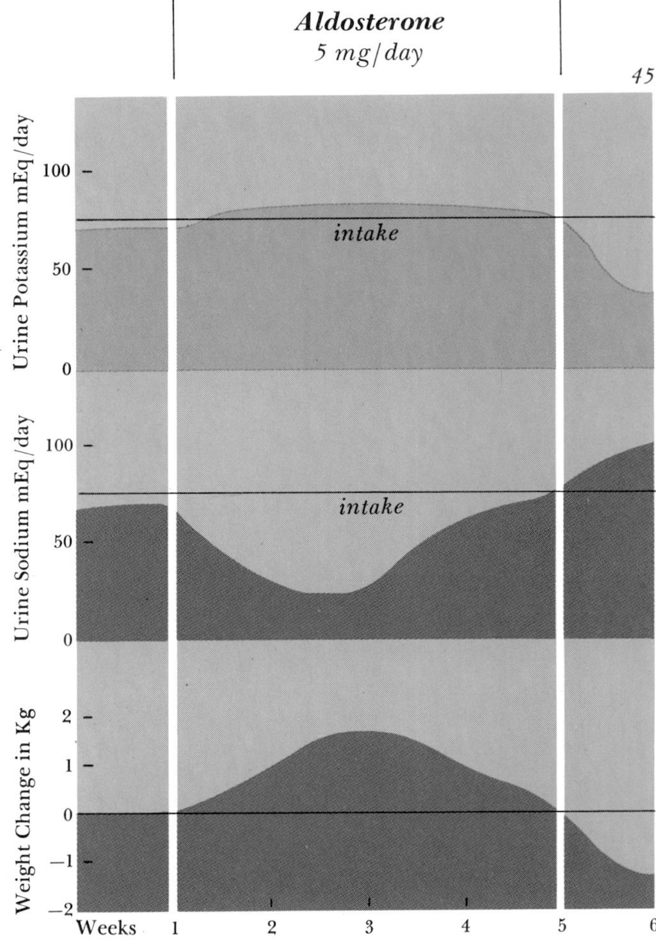

Synthetic Steroids

In attempts to improve the therapeutic effectiveness of the first used adrenal steroid, cortisone, by enhancing its anti-inflammatory properties and abolishing the adverse side effects, literally hundreds of synthetic steroid compounds have been synthesized and biologically tested. Relatively few compounds have been developed which, through increased potency, and dissociation of glucocorticoid from mineralocorticoid activity, or through decreased cost of production, have become useful drugs in the clinical practice of medicine. It should be realized that to date no attempt to separate one glucocorticoid effect from another has been successful. Moreover, the glucocorticoid action is directly related to its ACTH suppressing ability. It has, however, been possible to synthesize pure glucocorticoids and potent mineralocorticoids. The goal of producing potent anti-inflammatory steroids with no adverse effects has not yet been realized.

Steroid chemists have made structural modifications of the steroid molecule which alter action in one or several ways by: 1. Increasing the potency by increasing the resistance of the molecule to the normal metabolic inactivating systems of the liver; 2. Increasing the activity of the biologically important 11-OH group; 3. Altering the solubility and absorption rate of the steroid; 4. Altering the protein binding capacity of the steroid in the circulation.

Examples of the manner in which this has been accomplished are as follows: *(Fig. 47)*.

Introduction of a double bond at the 1-2 position in ring A increases the glucocorticoid potency of cortisol five times by making the △4-3 ketone group more inaccessible to enzymatic inactivation. The resultant substance, prednisolone (prednisone, if made from cortisone compounds) is used because its mineralocorticoid effect, compared to that of cortisol, was not increased. Substitution of a methyl group at C_6 has a similar effect.

9-α Halogenation. The addition of a fluoride atom at the 9-α position increases glucocorticoid activity considerably, but the mineralocorticoid activity of cortisol is also increased 300 times—making 9-α fluoro-hydrocortisone equal in mineralocorticoid potency to aldosterone. Since this drug is effective by mouth, in contrast to aldosterone, this is the mineralocorticoid of choice in the treatment of Addison's disease. It is thought that

Fig. 45 *Daily injections of aldosterone in a normal subject first lead to sodium and water retention with an increase in weight. Escape from this is illustrated by a leveling off in weight gain and a return of sodium excretion to equal intake. Note that the negative potassium balance continues.*

Fig. 46 *Molecular formulae showing the similarity of aldosterone to progesterone and spironolactone. Both substances impair the action of aldosterone at a distal tubular tissue receptor site by competitive inhibition.*

Aldosterone

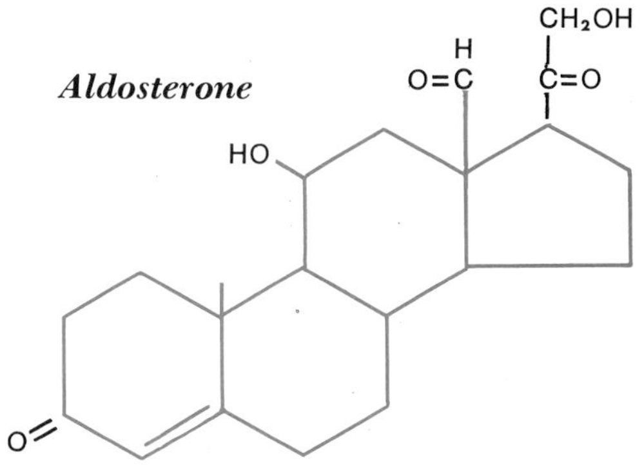

HO, H, O=C, CH_2OH, C=O, O=

Progesterone

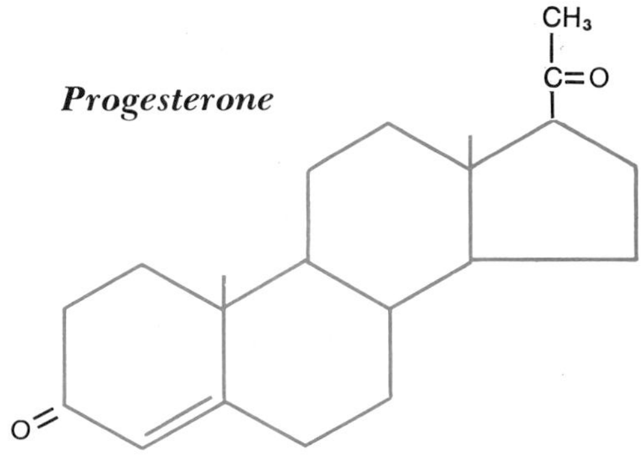

CH_3, C=O, O=

Spironolactone

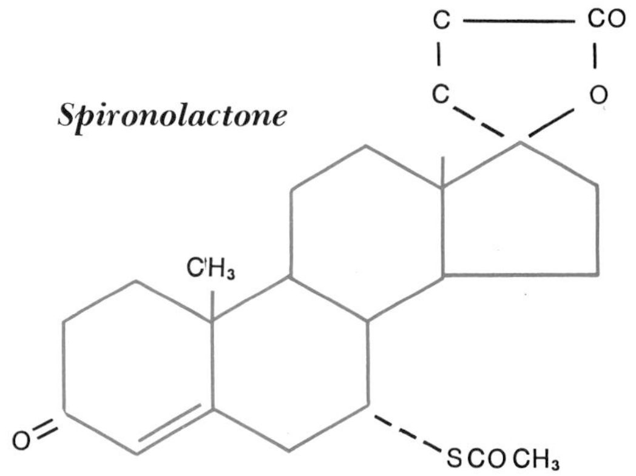

C, CO, C, O, CH_3, O=, $SCOCH_3$

Fig. 46

9-α halogen substitution prevents oxidation of the closely related 11β hydroxy group and/or hinders reduction of the A ring.

Introduction of an α methyl group at position 16 greatly enhances glucocorticoid activity by decreasing the rate of inactivation of the 20, 21 α-ketol side chain. If this substitution to cortisol is made in addition to the double bond at position 1 and the 9α fluorine substitution, the extremely potent glucocorticoid dexamethasone is produced. This synthetic steroid has negligible mineralocorticoid effect. Here reduction of the A ring is hindered by the 1-2 double bond, 11β-hydroxyl-oxidation is hindered by the 9α fluro substitution and side chain destruction is altered by the 16α methyl group. This compound has a half-life three to four times that of cortisol and is thirty times as potent in glucocorticoid activity. *(Fig. 48).*

All steroids with an 11-keto group must have this reduced to the 11-hydroxy group before the compound is biologically active as a glucocorticoid. This is accomplished by the liver. In a very few patients this conversion is not efficient and substances such as cortisone and prednisone, as compared to cortisol and prednisolone, are relatively inactive. In practice it is usually best to prescribe only the 11-hydroxylated steroids if an extremely serious illness is present or if a question of a lack of effective medication arises. In general, the cost of the two drugs is comparable.

47

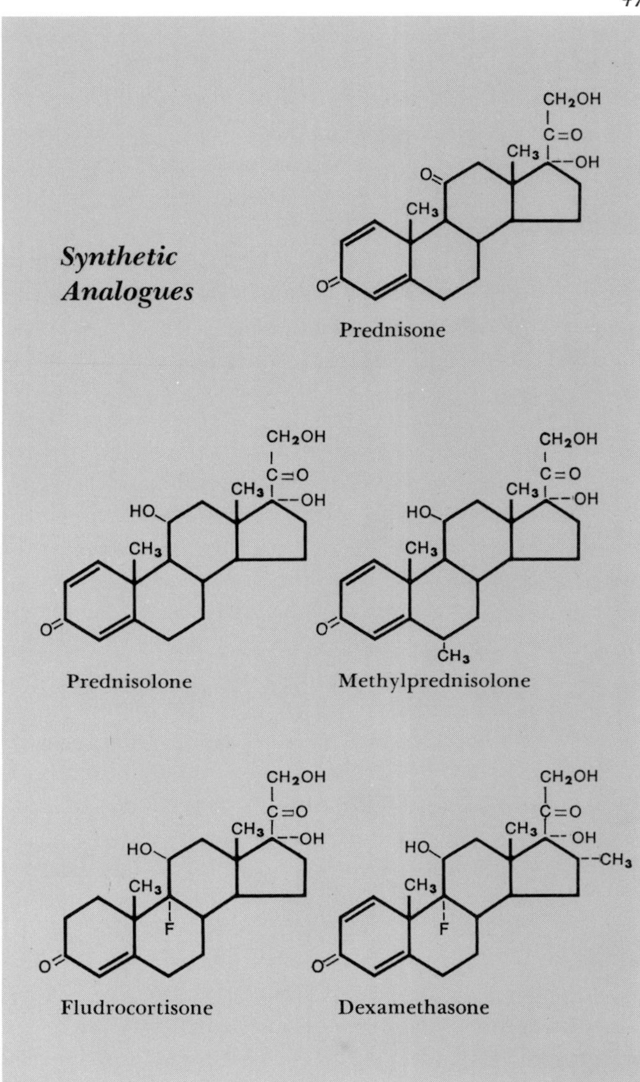

Fig. 47 *Synthetic analogues of glucocorticoids and mineralocorticoids used in medical practice.*

Fig. 48 *Relative glucocorticoid & mineralocorticoid potency and tablet strength of natural and synthetic adrenal steroids.*

48

Relative Potency and Tablet Size

Corticosteroid	*Glucocorticoid Activity*	*Mineralocorticoid Activity*	*Standard Tablet Strength*
Cortisol	1	1	20 mg
Cortisone	0.8	0.8	25 mg
Aldosterone	0.3	300	—
Corticosterone	0.5	1.5	—
Deoxycorticosterone	0	20	—
Prednisone	4	0.3	5 mg
Prednisolone	5	0.3	4 mg
Methylprednisolone	5	0	4 mg
Dexamethasone	30	0	0.75, 0.5 mg
Fludrocortisone	8	250	0.1 mg

5 Addison's Disease

Adrenocortical Insufficiency

Adrenocortical hormone secretion may be insufficient to maintain normal life because of: A) primary disease or dysfunction of the adrenal cortex, or B) deficient ACTH (secondary adrenal insufficiency).

Primary adrenal insufficiency may be classified as: *Addison's disease*—involves all zones of the cortex; *Hypoaldosteronism*—involves the zona glomerulosa only; or *Adrenogenital syndrome*—enzymatic defects occur in all three zones.

Secondary adrenal insufficiency may be classified as: *Pituitary or hypothalmic insufficiency* due to disease, trauma or surgery; or *Iatrogenic pituitary insufficiency* due to exogenous steroid treatment.

Addison's Disease

Incidence: Addison's disease may be found in four persons per 100,000 population. It occurs equally in both sexes when due to tuberculosis and is more common in adults than children. Idiopathic atrophy is more common in females and children.

Pathology: Over 90% of primary adrenal insufficiency is caused by (1) bilateral tuberculosis of the adrenal glands, or (2) bilateral atrophy of unknown etiology.

It may also be caused by bilateral involvement of the

Fig. 49 *Cross-sections of an adrenal gland involved by tuberculosis. Note the large size of the gland and the absence of an identifiable medulla.*

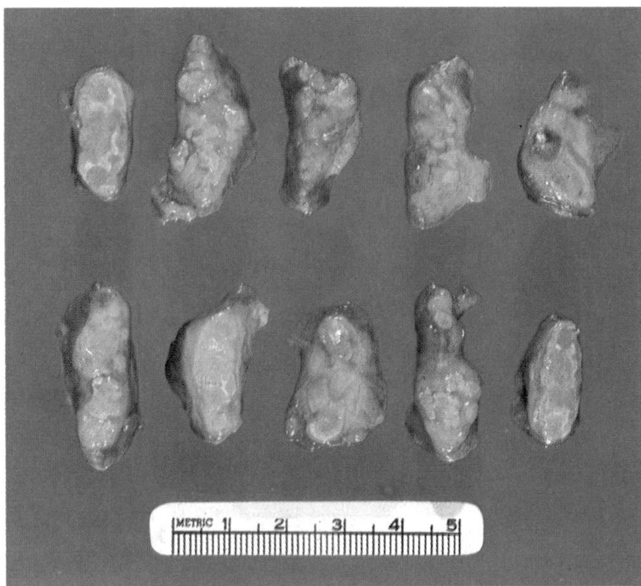

50

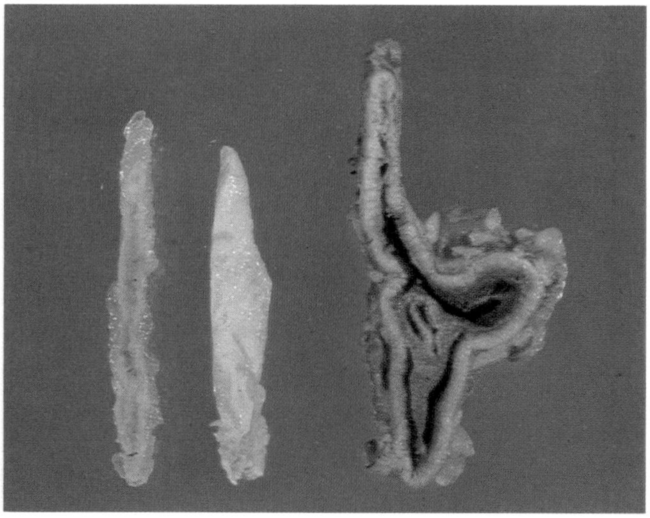

51

Disorders
associated with Addison's Disease in an unexpectedly high frequency

- Diabetes Mellitus
- Pernicious Anemia
- Idiopathic hypoparathyroidism
- Thyrotoxicosis
- Spontaneous myxedema
- Hachimoto's thyroiditis
- Primary gonadal failure
- Diffuse cerebral sclerosis (Schilder's disease)
- Superficial moniliasis

adrenal glands in amyloidosis, blastomycosis, coccidioidomycosis, histoplasmosis, lymphomas and leukemic infiltrations, bilateral adrenal hemorrhage, and very rarely with bilateral metastatic tumor. Although metastatic infiltration of the adrenal glands is common in end stage carcinoma, it is exceedingly rare for this to produce adrenal insufficiency. Usually well over 80% of both glands must be destroyed before signs and symptoms of insufficiency develop.

In most reports idiopathic atrophy is now slightly more common than tuberculosis as a cause of Addison's disease. Tuberculosis involves the medulla as well as the cortex with nodular caseations. *(Fig. 49)* In idiopathic atrophy, the entire cortex is reduced to a fibrous remnant surrounding the intact medulla. *(Fig. 50)* The induction of hypoglycemia, a well known stimulus to epinephrine release from the adrenal medulla, will therefore increase blood and urine epinephrine in the patient with Addison's disease due to idiopathic atrophy and not in the patient with tuberculosis. This has been suggested as a clinical test for differentiating atrophy from tuberculosis. In idiopathic atrophy circulating antibodies to adrenal tissue occur in the majority of patients. This suggests an autoimmune cause for the atrophy. Similar antibody titers are not found in patients with tuberculosis. Although adrenal tuberculosis is usually secondary to infection in another organ, the latter may not always be readily evident for there may be a very long latent period between the primary tuberculous infection and the development of adrenal insufficiency.

A familial occurrence of adrenal atrophy has been reported. An association with other endocrine organ autoimmune disease is conspicuous. *(Fig. 51)* These diseases have many common associations which group them with autoimmune phenomena. They occur more frequently in females and in families; they have organ-specific antibodies in the serum and histologically are characterized by lymphocytic infiltration and atrophy. However, despite all this, an autoimmune *cause* for adrenal atrophy has yet to be proven.

Fig. 50 *Adrenal gland from a normal subject on the right. On the left is the adrenal gland found at post mortem in a patient with Addison's disease due to adrenal atrophy. Note the central core of medullary tissue remains intact.*

Fig. 51 *List of disorders associated with Addison's disease in an unexpectedly high frequency.*

Fig. 52 *Addisonian pigmentation may be difficult to discern in the negro. Note the increased pigmentation on the face, hands and forearm (areas exposed to light) and the increased pigmentation around the scar below the left breast.*

Fig. 53 *Frequency of signs and symptoms in patients with Addison's disease.*

Fig. 54 *Relationship of the signs and symptoms in Addison's disease to glucocorticoid or mineralocorticoid deficiency.*

Clinical Manifestations

Chronic Adrenal Insufficiency—Addison's Disease: Thomas Addison's original description of the presentation of chronic adrenal insufficiency cannot be bettered. In 1855 he wrote: "The leading and characteristic features of the morbid state to which I would direct attention are anemia, general languor and debility, remarkable feebleness of the heart's action, irritability of the stomach, and a peculiar change of colour in the skin, occurring in connection with a diseased condition of the suprarenal capsules." *(Fig. 53)*

The diagnosis is usually suspected because of weakness and tiredness in a patient with hypotension and darkly pigmented skin.

Pigmentation and weakness are almost essential to consideration of the diagnosis. Both are due to glucocorticoid insufficiency. *(Fig. 54)* In the absence of cortisol, ACTH and β-MSH in blood rise to exceedingly high concentrations. β-MSH stimulates melanophore activity creating the typical tan with darkened mucosal membranes and conspicuous moles. *(Fig. 52)* This is not due to ACTH. Both regress with proper replacement therapy and the skin will lighten considerably with time, although it is rare to have it return completely to normal. In some patients the initial darkly tanned skin will later develop vitiliginous white patches. *(Fig. 55)*

Disturbance of gastrointestinal function is a common presenting complaint. It may vary from mild anorexia

53

Frequency
of signs and symptoms
in Addison's Disease

Sign or Symptom	*Occurrence %*
Weakness	99
Pigmentation	98
Weight Loss	97
Hypotension	90
Anorexia	90
Vomiting	84
Nausea	81
Abdominal Pain	34
Constipation	28
Salt Craving	22
Diarrhoea	21
Syncope	16
Vitiligo	9

52

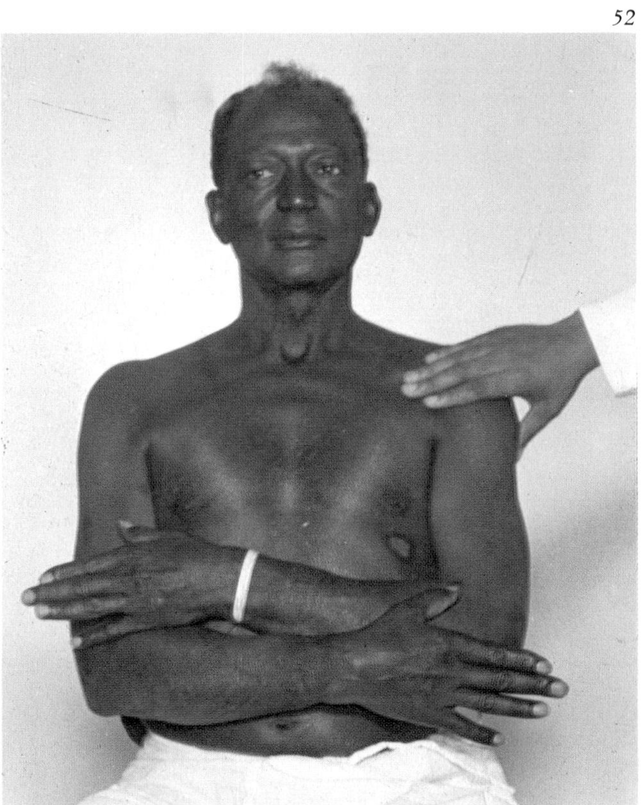

54

Signs and Symptoms
in Addison's Disease as related
to glucocorticoid or
mineralocorticoid deficiency

Mineralocorticoid deficiency	*Glucocorticoid deficiency*
hypotension	weakness
hyponatremia	fatigue
lethargy	weight loss
easy fatigue	hypoglycemia
virtigo	pigmentation
syncope	water metabolism
	irritability
	mental sluggishness
	increased sensitivity to taste

to nausea or pain severe enough to present an "acute surgical abdomen". *(Fig. 56-63)*

Electrolyte Abnormalities: In chronic adrenocortical failure, the absence of both glucocorticoid and mineralocorticoid activity leads to dehydration and body fluid compartment contraction. Blood volume falls as sodium is lost through the kidney; potassium and nitrogen excretion is impaired. The typical serum chemistry of primary adrenal insufficiency is a decreased serum sodium concentration, an increased serum potassium concentration and an increased BUN. Occasionally, with severe adrenal insufficiency serum calcium is found to be slightly elevated.

Hematologic Abnormalities: In chronic adrenal insufficiency the hemoconcentration present may mask an underlying mild anemia, usually of the iron-deficiency type. This may become noticeable as hydration occurs with treatment. In some patients, macrocytic anemia occurs in association with antibodies for intrinsic factor, supporting a long held opinion that Addisonian pernicious anemia and Addison's disease may be related.

X-Ray Findings in Addison's Disease: 1. Calcification of the cartilage of the ear ("stiff ears") and of the costal cartilage may be seen in some patients with adrenal insufficiency. 2. The heart is small in size in uncomplicated adrenal insufficiency. 3. Calcification of the adrenal glands is observed in a minority of patients with granulomatous disease.

Acute Adrenal Insufficiency—Addisonian Crisis: The abrupt cessation of replacement therapy in a well treated patient with Addison's disease or the challenge of a stress, such as infection, trauma or surgery in a patient with chronic adrenal insufficiency may precipitate a crisis and lead to death. It is usually manifest by weakness, syncope, hypotension, rapidly progressing with hyperpyrexia to vascular collapse, shock and death. Costovertebral or abdominal pain may be present. The course may be so rapid that no electrolyte changes occur. Diagnosis is made on clinical signs and symptoms and the response of the patient to an infusion of 100 mg of intravenous hydrocortisone combined with the usual restorative procedures for shock and dehydration. There is no contraindication to such a clinical trial in the gravely ill patient. Blood pressure will usually respond within one-half to two hours and if no response is seen in eight hours, the diagnosis of adrenal insufficiency is very unlikely.

Diagnosis: The diagnosis of Addison's disease is confirmed by demonstrating a functional inability of the adrenal cortex to respond to ACTH. Since there is a great overlap between low and normal plasma and urine values for cortisol and cortisol metabolites, it is useless to measure them in the basal state. Many modifications of standard tests have been used. Most are acceptable. The following is convenient: 0.25 mg of

55

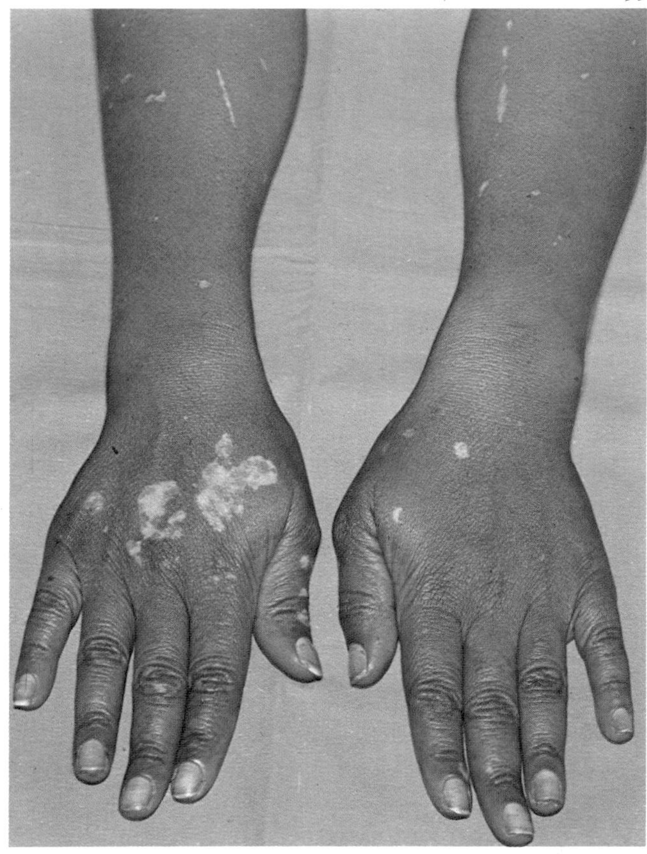

56

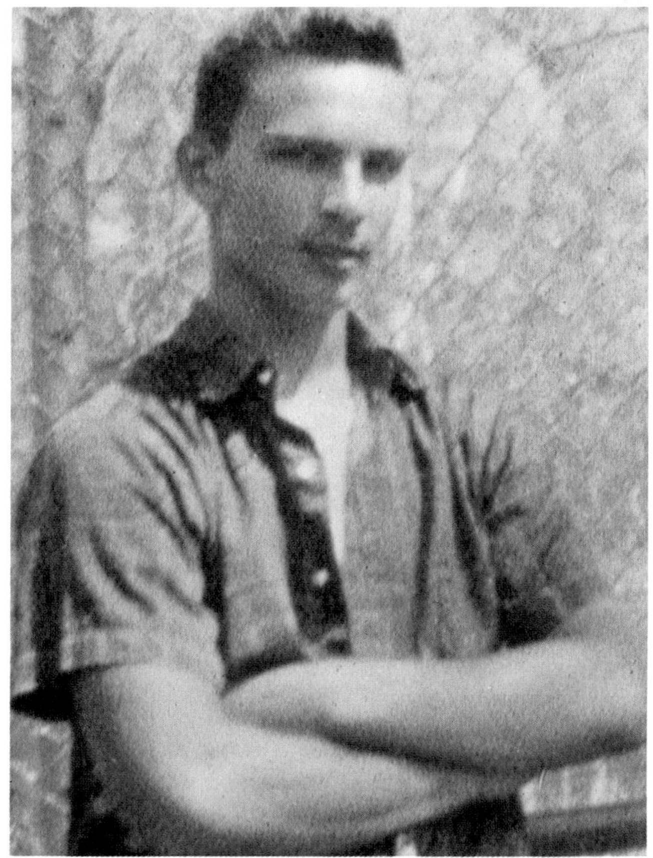

Fig. 55 Vitiligo appearing on the hands of a patient with mild, but chronic Addisonian pigmentation.

Fig. 56 Picture of a patient with Addison's disease two years before diagnosis.

Fig. 57 Same patient (Fig. 56) at the time of diagnosis. Note the marked increase in pigmentation despite the poor quality of the previous picture.

Fig. 58 Hands of a patient with Addison's disease showing the typical pigment collection in the palmar creases.

Fig. 59 Increased pigmentation at the edge of a recently healed scar in this patient. (Fig. 57)

Fig. 60 Typical site of pigmentation on lips and gums.(Fig. 57)

Fig. 61 Close-up of the pigmentation showing discreet melanin clumping. (Fig. 57)

58

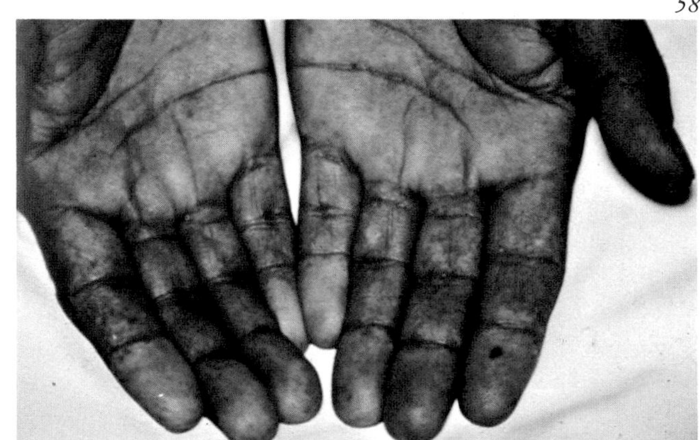

59

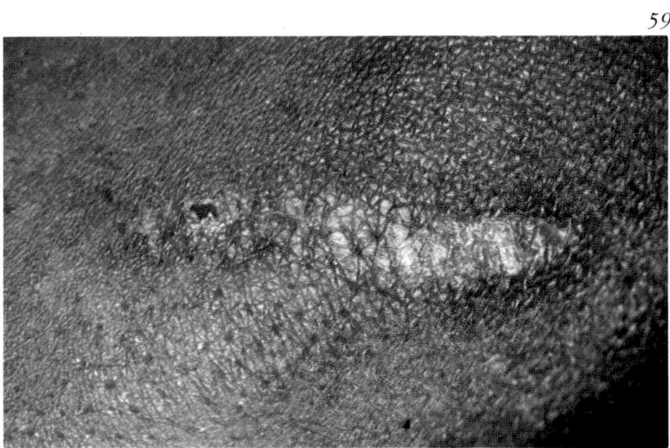

57

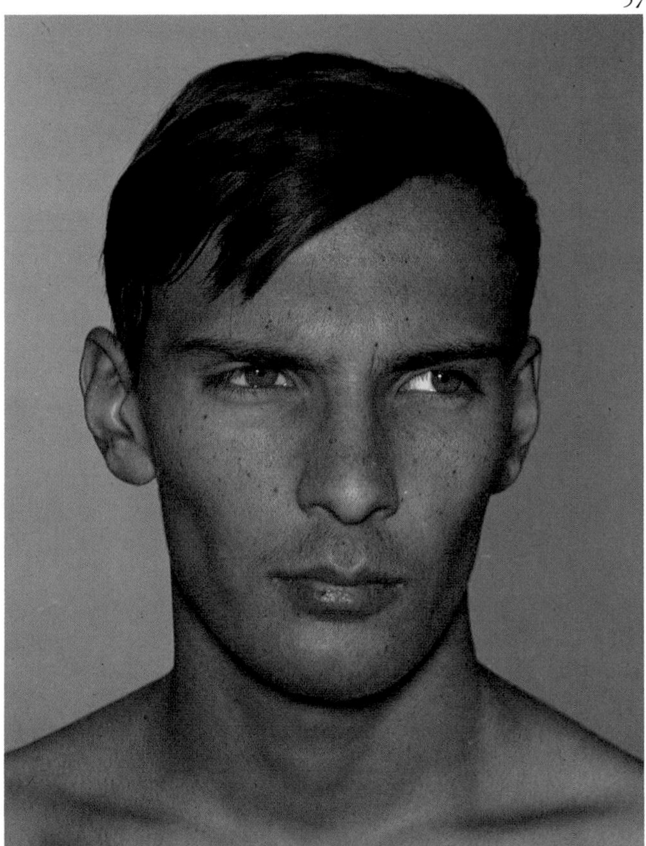

60

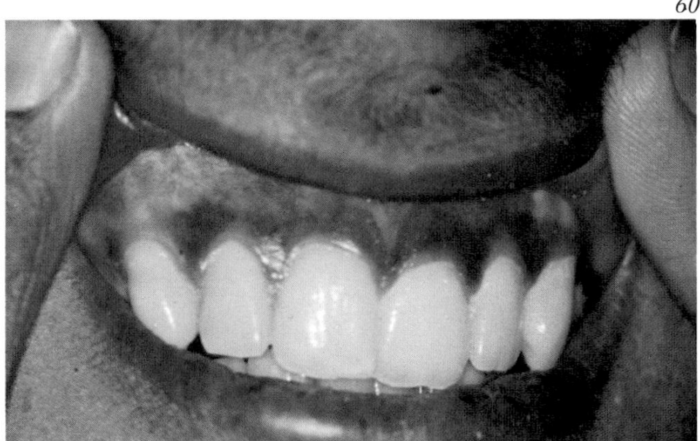

61

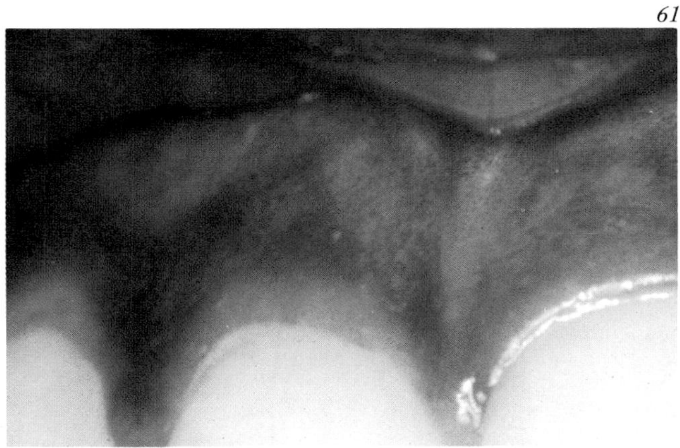

synthetic ACTH is infused by vein over an eight-hour period. Plasma cortisol is measured at the beginning and end. If an increase of over 20 mg/100 ml is found, Addison's disease is not present. The plasma concentration is usually less than 5 mg/100 ml and does not change with the infusion in true Addison's disease.

Frequently, the diagnosis is suspected by the physician but not seriously enough to warrant hospitalization. In such cases it is sufficient to give a single dose of 0.25 mg of synthetic ACTH intravenously and collect blood for cortisol one hour later. If cortisol concentration is greater than 8 mg%, the diagnosis is ruled out.

Secondary Adrenal Insufficiency: In the complete absence of ACTH, the human adrenal cortex begins to atrophy in one week. This secondary adrenal insufficiency may be caused by disease of the pituitary gland and hypothalamus or by ACTH suppression due to exogenous glucocorticoid administration. Steroid suppression is without a doubt the commonest cause of adrenal insufficiency.

Pituitary-Hypothalamic Insufficiency: The adrenal insufficiency observed is usually associated with deficiency of other pituitary hormones, but occasionally it is due to an isolated loss of ACTH. In panhypopituitarism, signs of adrenal failure are usually mild until the patient is severely stressed, when mental confusion and signs of vascular collapse may occur apparently without sufficient cause. In this instance the patient would not be pigmented, and in fact, may be even somewhat underpigmented. The serum sodium would be low and the BUN and serum potassium would be in the normal range, as contrasted to primary adrenal insufficiency, for the intact renin angiotensin system maintains a relatively adequate aldosterone secretion rate. The glucocorticoid loss, in the presence of a normal aldosterone effect, leads to water retention rather than to dehydration and the symptoms are related more to water intoxication than to water dehydration. A small dose of cortisol rapidly leads to a water diuresis and restores the patient to normal. This syndrome must be distinguished from the inappropriate ADH syndrome in which cortisol has no such effect.

The diagnosis is confirmed by demonstrating deficiency of other pituitary hormones, such as thyroid stimulating hormone, growth hormone or gonadotrophins. Direct stimulation of both ACTH and growth hormone may be achieved by the insulin stimulation test; 0.15 units of crystalline insulin per kg of body weight is given to produce a fall in blood sugar to below 40 mg/100 ml. A serum growth hormone and cortisol determination one hour after the injection should both increase significantly (GH greater than 10 mg/ml, cortisol, greater than 20 mg/100 ml).

If the results of either of the above are equivocal, a metyrapone test should be done. This test can be performed in one of two ways, the standard two-day test or the overnight administration of metyrapone.

The standard two-day test: The patient is given 750 mg of metyrapone every four hours for two days. Urinary 17-hydroxysteroid or ketogenic steroids are measured for a control day, on the last day and the day after this dose. There should be a doubling of the steroids if the adrenal pituitary activity is normal.

Overnight stimulation: A single dose of metyrapone (30 mg per kg of body weight) is given with a glass of milk at 12 midnight. Blood ACTH and 11-deoxycortisol measurements are made on samples withdrawn at

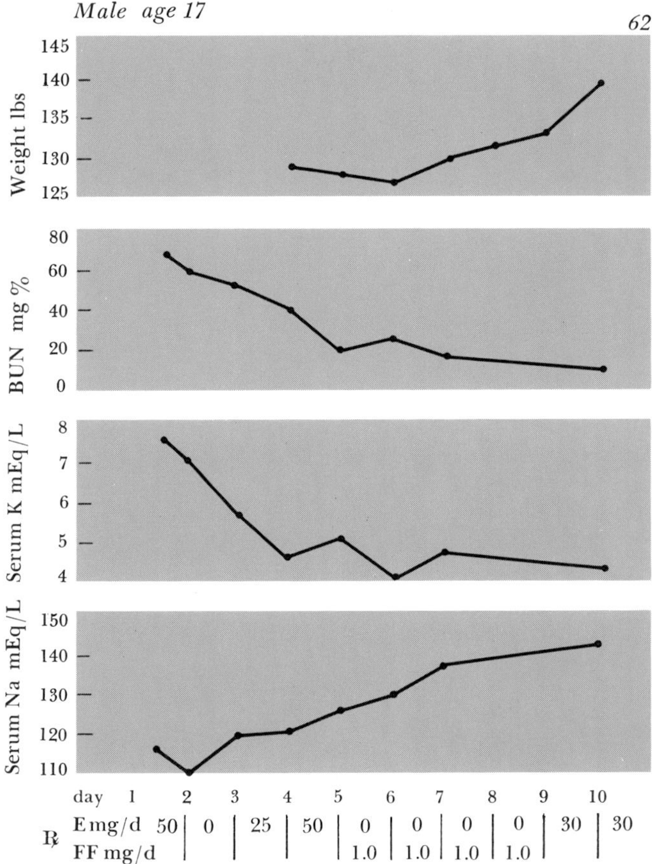

Fig. 62 *Chart of the initial serum electrolytes found in patient in Figure 57 on admission to hospital. Treatment with small amounts of cortisone (E) led to rapid restoration of these abnormalities. On days five to nine, cortisone treatment was discontinued and fludrocortisone (FF), was substituted in order to perform the tests shown on the control days.*

Fig. 63 *The high level of 17 ketogenic steroids were the metabolites of the administrated cortisone. No adrenal steroid response occurred during three days of intravenous* ACTH *infusion. Plasma cortisol did not rise above 3 µg %. In this patient an additional study, showing that the small amount of 17 ketosteroids found were produced by the testes, was demonstrated by the administration of ethinylestradiol over five days. Gonadotroph suppression by the estrogen caused the 17 ketosteroid excretion to fall, indicating the gonad origin of these steroids in this patient with Addison's disease.*

8 a.m. If these determinations are not available, urine is collected for twenty-four hours for 17-hydroxycorticosteroid or 17-ketogenic steroid determinations. If the patient is normal, plasma deoxycortisol should be greater than 8 μg/100 ml and plasma ACTH over 200 μg/ml. Urinary deoxycortical steroids, as measured by the 17-hydroxy steroid or the 17-ketogenic steroid methods should be greater than 6 mg/24 hours and 10 mg/24 hours, respectively.

Treatment

Chronic adrenal insufficiency: The therapeutic aim is to restore the patient to normal by substituting the equivalent quantities of cortisol and mineralocorticoid by mouth for the usual daily output of the adrenal of these steroids. The dose of cortisol varies from 15 to 30 mg and is usually administered in one or two doses per day, two-thirds being given in the morning and one-third late in the afternoon. Since aldosterone is ineffective by mouth because of its rapid inactivation by the liver, fludrocortisone, a mineralocorticoid of potency equal to aldosterone, is given by mouth in a dose of 0.1 mg/day. The dose of cortisol is gauged by weight gain and sense of well being of the patient. Beginning therapy is occasionally associated with a voracious appetite, a rapid gain in weight and mild sleeplessness. The dose should be reduced; weight gain can usually be controlled by diet therapy. At monthly visits, the patient's weight and blood pressure should be taken and the ankles checked for edema. If the blood pressure rises, in association with a mild gain in weight, or with mild edema, the dose of fludrocortisone should be reduced. Occasionally, the dose may be decreased to 0.05 mg or in some patients occasionally increased to 0.2 mg. The small dose may be given every other day to a patient with mild heart failure. Pharmacologic side effects are rarely encountered at these small replacement doses.

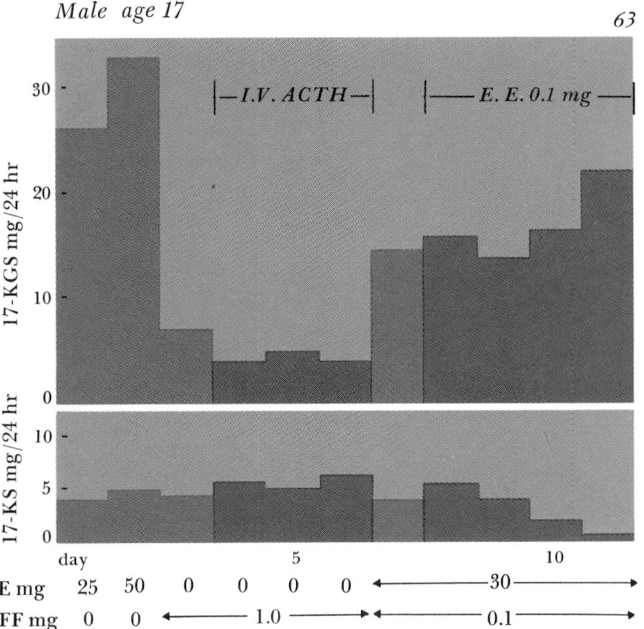

A patient receiving long-term steroid therapy should be instructed to double the dose of cortisol in the presence of a mild upper respiratory infection. If a fever of 100-101° is present, the dose should be tripled and the patient should be seen immediately by a physician. If there is any reason to suspect that the illness is serious, the patient should be hospitalized. In a well-controlled Addisonian patient, this does not often occur.

Acute adrenal insufficiency: Acute adrenal insufficiency should be immediately treated by the infusion of 100 mg of intravenous hydrocortisone dissolved in a small amount of saline. This is followed by 100 mg of intravenous hydrocortisone dissolved in 1 liter of isotonic saline to be infused over the following eight hours. This is in addition to replacement by 1 to 2 liters of normal saline as required to restore blood volumes; 100 mg of hydrocortisone is then given intravenously over the following 15 hours, again dissolved in normal saline. Because of the large amounts of saline given, it is unnecessary to give mineralocorticoid. Hydrocortisone is prescribed in divided doses three or four times a day by mouth or intramuscularly until the patient has returned to the normal maintenance dosage, usually within four or five days.

Iatrogenic adrenocortical insufficiency: Long-term glucocorticoid treatment at ACTH suppressive doses for over a week may lead to functional adrenocortical atrophy. Such patients, when stressed by infection, trauma or surgery, are unable to respond with the usual increased output of cortisol of up to 200 or 300 mg per day. Proper management aims to mimic the normal response. Since there is a lag of about 1 to 2 hours in glucocorticoid effect, the patient about to undergo major surgery should receive 100 mg of hydrocortisone intramuscularly two hours before the induction of anesthesia. Alternatively, an infusion of 100 mg of intravenous hydrocortisone dissolved in 500 ml of 5% glucose and water is begun two hours before surgery and continued up to the time of induction of anesthesia. Another 100 mg is given by vein throughout surgery and followed by 100 mg during the remainder of the twenty-four hour period. The dose is halved each day until the normal replacement dosage is reached by the fourth or fifth postoperative day.

If the surgical procedure is minor, 100 mg of parenteral hydrocortisone is given two hours prior to anesthetic induction and 100 mg is then continued through the rest of the day. For minor surgery under local anesthesia 50-100 mg of hydrocortisone may be given by mouth two hours before the procedure. If trauma has occurred or an emergency arises, the patient should be treated as though acute adrenal crisis has occurred in an Addisonian patient.

6 Cushing's Syndrome

64

Anatomic
Bilateral adrenal hyperplasia
Adrenal adenoma
Adrenal carcinoma
Nodular adrenal hyperplasia
Ectopic ACTH secreting neoplasm

Pathophysiologic
Pituitary dependent
Pituitary independent
a. Adrenal tumor
b. Ectopic tumor

In 1932 Dr. Harvey Cushing described twelve cases of a disorder, which he suggested was due to "pituitary-basophilism," even though basophilic tumors were found in only three of the twelve cases, and in spite of the fact that one case had a well defined adrenal adenoma. Since a careful study of these cases suggests multiple causes of the syndrome, the eponym Cushing's syndrome has come to mean the clinical entity due to excessive and prolonged action of glucocorticoids. Since glucocorticoids are commonly used drugs, the clinical appearance of hypercortisolism is generally familiar to all physicians.

A pathophysiologic classification of the causes of Cushing's syndrome is as follows: *(Fig. 64)*. *Adrenocortical hyperplasia due to;* a) excess pituitary ACTH, b) excess ACTH from ectopic non-endocrine tumors. *Adrenal tumor due to;* a) adrenal cortical adenoma, b) adrenal cortical carcinoma. *Iatrogenic;* a) ACTH administration, b) glucocorticoid medication.

Cushing's syndrome is not a common disease, occurring in approximately one in five thousand hospital admissions. It is three to four times as common in females as males and occurs most frequently between the ages of 25 and 35. Before the advent of a satisfactory form of treatment for this condition, death usually occurred within five years of the onset of symptoms.

The clinical description by Dr. Cushing included most of the features currently associated with florid cortisol excess. In the severe case, most of the adverse effects of glucocorticoids previously enumerated are found. The characteristic features *(Fig. 65)* include truncal and facial obesity in the presence of thin extremities (central obesity), the "moonface" is often plethoric and associated with hypertension, purple striae, weakness, and in females, acne and hirsutism. Once seen, the typical "Cushingoid" appearance of hypercortisolism is not soon forgotten. *(Fig. 66)* However, it is the aim of modern practice to make the diagnosis before florid signs and symptoms are present. The most valuable early signs are the rounded face, hypertension and some evidence of hirsutism, such as increased hair growth, acne or menstrual irregularities and the presence of rather thin skin on the extremities, perhaps with easy bruisability. *(Fig. 67-69)* When these appear in a female of child bearing age, the diagnosis of Cushing's

66

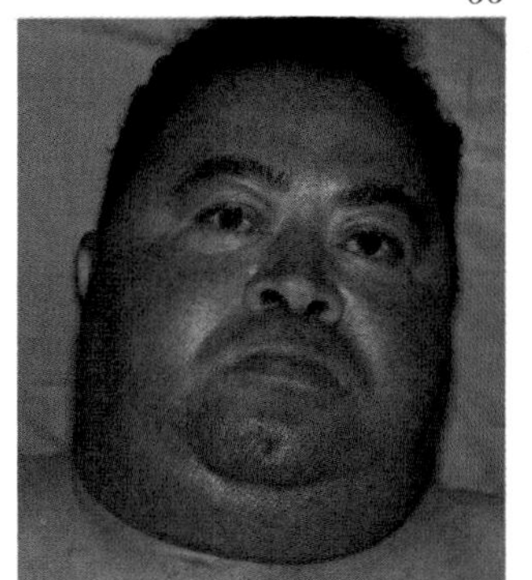

67

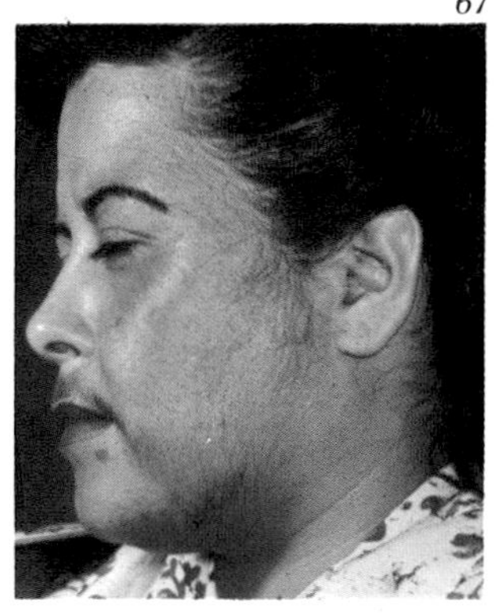

Fig. 64 *Etiology of Cushing's syndrome.*

Fig. 65 *Cushing's syndrome, signs and symptoms.*

Fig. 66 *Classic facial features observed in a patient with Cushing's syndrome.*

Fig. 67 *Hirsutism in a female patient with Cushing's syndrome manifested primarily as androgen excess.*

Fig. 68 *Abdominal striae in a patient with Cushing's syndrome due to an adrenal adenoma.*

Fig. 69 *Lateral view of the same patient (Fig. 68) showing the marked trunkal obesity with thin arms and legs, the "centripetal obesity" characteristic of Cushing's syndrome.*

65

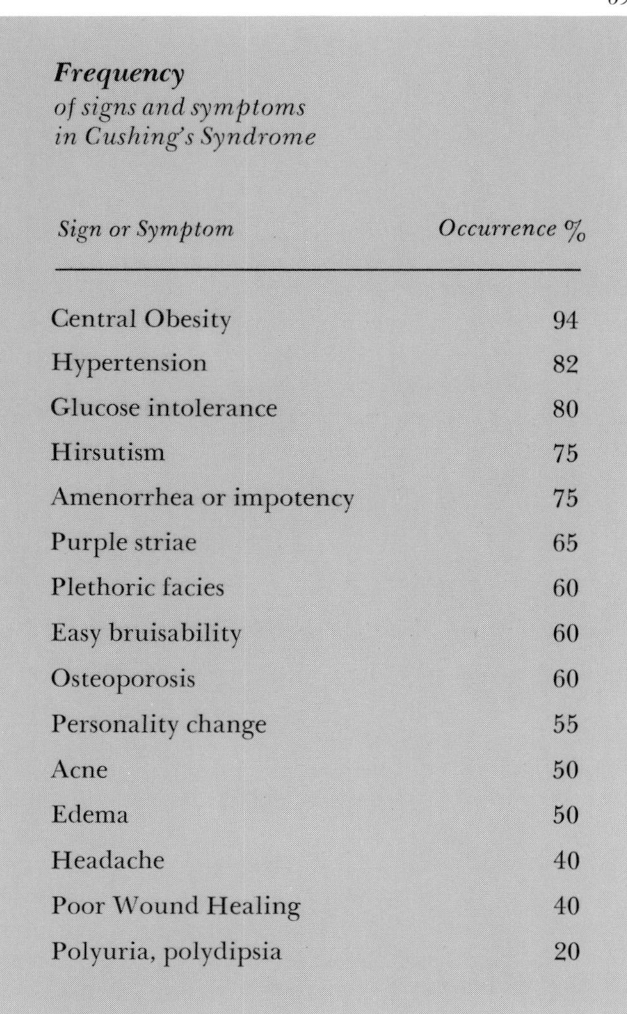

Frequency
of signs and symptoms
in Cushing's Syndrome

Sign or Symptom	*Occurrence %*
Central Obesity	94
Hypertension	82
Glucose intolerance	80
Hirsutism	75
Amenorrhea or impotency	75
Purple striae	65
Plethoric facies	60
Easy bruisability	60
Osteoporosis	60
Personality change	55
Acne	50
Edema	50
Headache	40
Poor Wound Healing	40
Polyuria, polydipsia	20

68

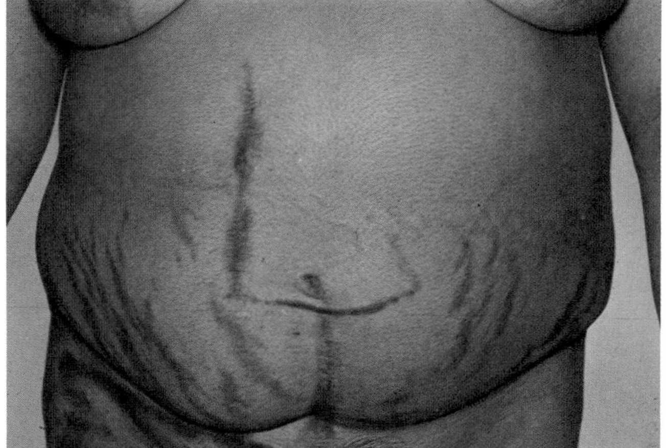

69

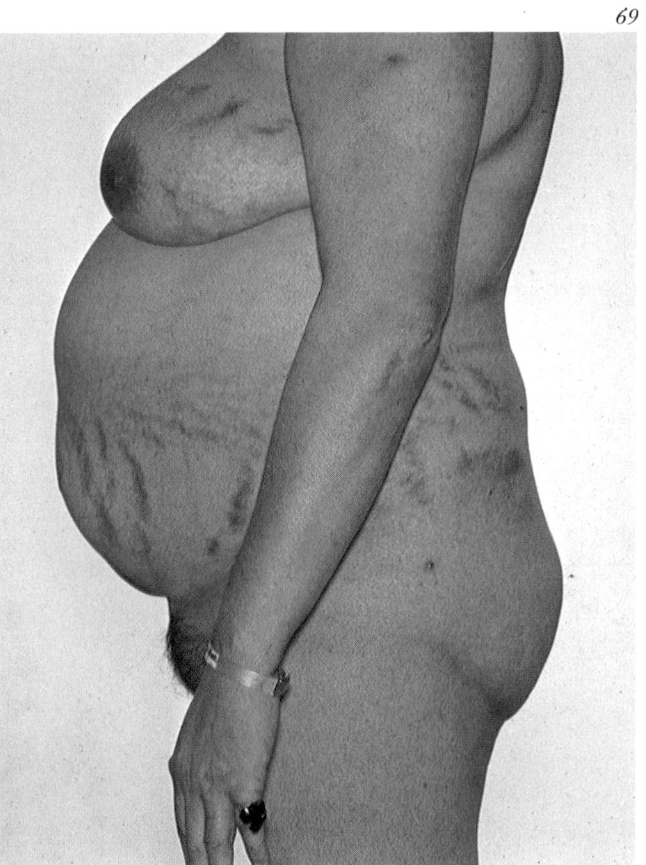

Fig. 70 *Series of pictures of a patient who had recurrent Cushing's syndrome following partial adrenalectomy. The large picture, taken two years after last postadrenalectomy photograph, demonstrates the return to normal following removal of the remnant tissue.*

Fig. 71a,b *Hyperplasia of the adrenal cortex. a) Glands removed surgically from a woman with Cushing's syndrome—combined weight 30 grams. b) Cross section reveals diffuse and nodular thickening of the cortex in both adrenals.*

Fig. 72 *Serum* ACTH *and urinary steroid response to pituitary suppression by dexamethasone and stimulation by metyrapone in a patient with Cushing's syndrome due to adrenal hyperplasia, as compared to the same tests performed in a normal subject. This clearly shows that the "set" of the glucocorticoid receptor mechanism is capable of responding to both decreased and increased serum cortisol concentration in this type of Cushing's syndrome. Note that the absolute level of* ACTH *is excessive.*

Fig. 73 *Adrenocortical adenoma attached to an atrophied adrenal gland. The color is typical.*

71a

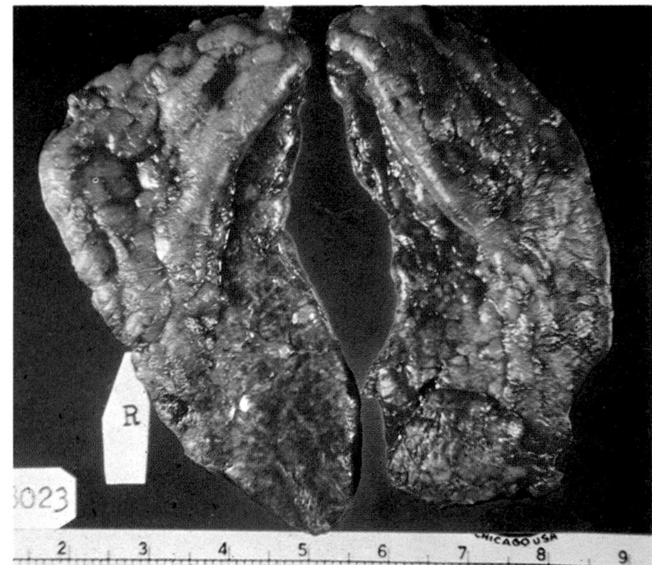

71b

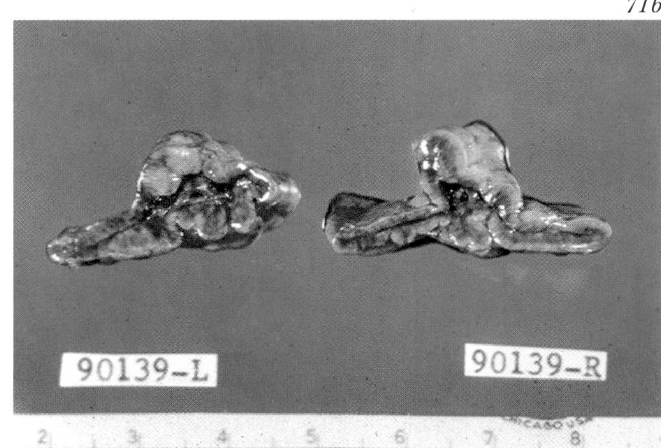

70

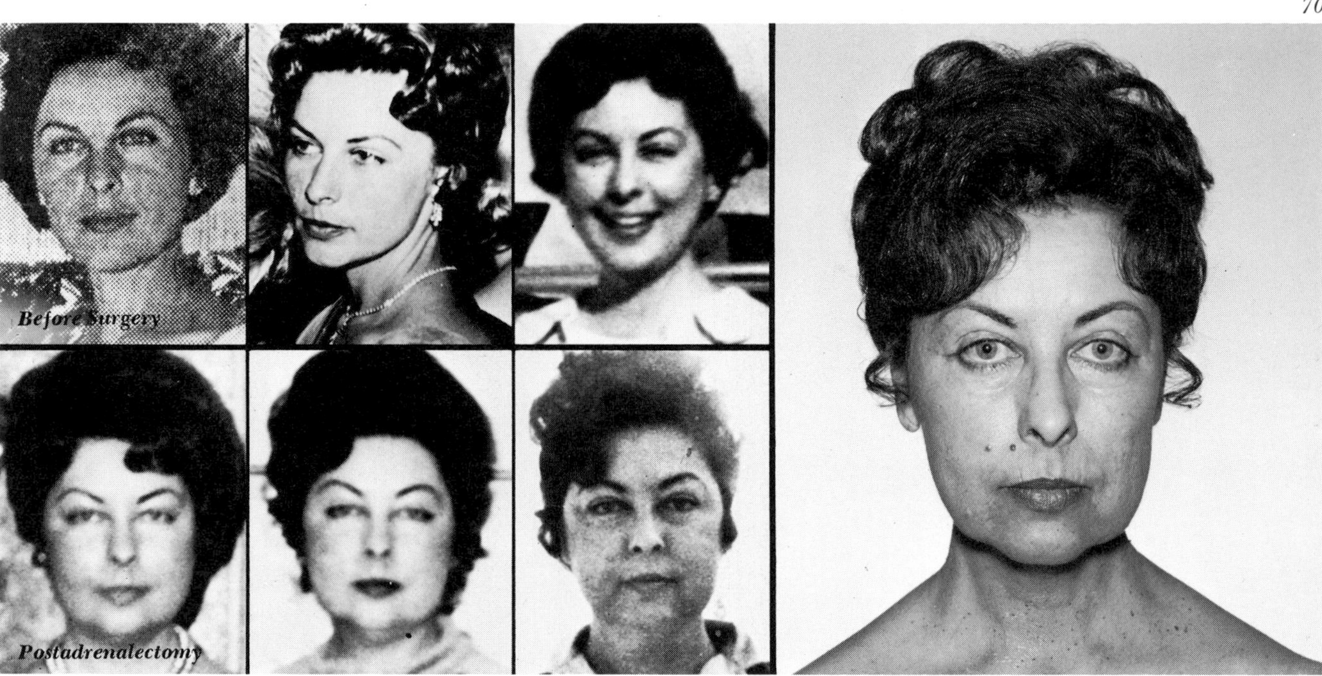

syndrome must be seriously considered. Of great value is the comparison of the patient's appearance with pictures taken some years earlier. *(Fig. 70)* The most frequent problem in the diagnosis occurs in the early stages of the syndrome when the patient may present only as a fat hairy girl with menstrual irregularities. More often than not, this is the final diagnosis, and not Cushing's syndrome, since simple obesity may be associated with mild hirsutism and with abnormalities of steroid metabolism. It is important to make this distinction and that requires the utilization of a knowledge of steroid dynamics in the various types of Cushing's syndrome.

Excess Pituitary ACTH Syndrome. Adrenocortical hyperplasia, secondary to excess ACTH is the cause of 75% of cases of Cushing's syndrome. *(Fig. 71)* In this common form of Cushing's syndrome, an abnormality of the hypothalamic-central nervous system neuroregulatory mechanism controlling the normal negative feedback of cortisol and ACTH secretion occurs. Early in Cushing's syndrome, plasma cortisol concentrations may be normal, but the normal diurnal reduction in cortisol secretion in the afternoon and evening is lost. Later, the plasma cortisol concentration may be elevated throughout the twenty-four hours. Despite this, the neuroregulatory receptors respond to stress, such as hypoglycemia or to a deficiency of cortisol (metopirone) by secreting increased ACTH and to suppression by high doses of glucocorticoid by decreasing pituitary release of ACTH. *(Fig. 72)* In a real sense this may be primary disease of the median eminence leading to hypercortisolism, because the number of ACTH bursts occurs more frequently throughout the day. Bilateral adrenal hyperplasia is the result. The primary abnormality of ACTH secretion is followed by an increased twenty-four hour secretion rate of cortisol by the adrenal glands.

Ectopic ACTH. A few non-endocrine malignant tumors have such altered DNA metabolism that a polypeptide substance, immunologically and biologically similar to pituitary ACTH, is produced and leads to bilateral adrenal hyperplasia and hypercortisolism. Carcinoma of the lung, thymus and kidney are the most frequently observed tumors. Since the tumors are usually inefficient at producing the peptide, the tumor is often large and conspicuous before manifestations of Cushing's syndrome appear. By then the toxic effects of the tumor usually produce a loss of weight and not the gain in weight seen in other forms of Cushing's syndrome. Often the clinical signs of Cushing's syndrome are slight, yet the cortisol secretion rate, plasma cortisol concentration and urinary cortisol metabolites are excessively high and give rise to typical hypokalemic alkalosis in the absence of the clinical appearance of Cushing's syndrome. This tumorous source of ACTH is relatively free of stimulatory or suppressant control by stress, glucocorticoid insufficiency or excess, as contrasted to Cushing's syndrome, due to the pituitary excess ACTH syndrome.

Adrenal Tumor. Benign adrenal cortical adenoma is found in 10 to 15% of patients with Cushing's syndrome. *(Fig. 73)* Adrenal carcinoma is causative in only 5 to 10%. The adrenal adenoma is bilateral in less than 10% of cases and is occasionally associated with hyperplasia—so-called adenomatous hyperplasia. Both tumors secrete adrenocortical steroids independent of the pituitary and usually therefore display no diurnal variation

72

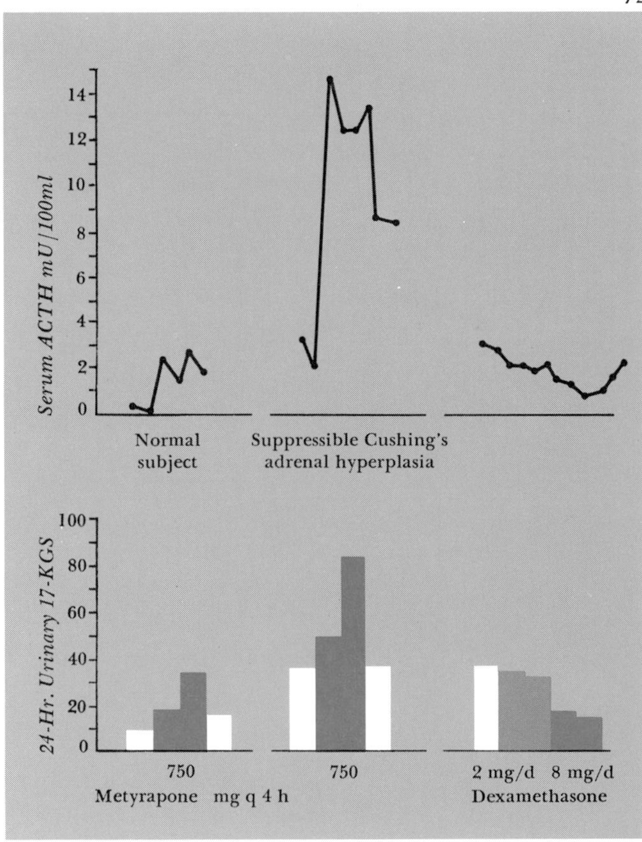

73

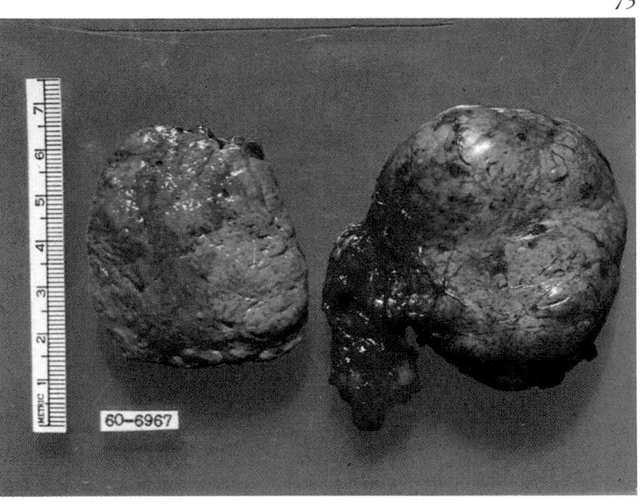

in serum cortisol. Moreover, pituitary ACTH release is suppressed for such a long time before diagnosis that the ACTH releasing system becomes functionally atrophied. This leads to atrophy of the adrenal tissue of the contralateral adrenal cortex and the adrenal cortex in the gland from which the tumor arose. These facts have great importance in establishing a cause for Cushing's syndrome, once the presence of hypercortisolism is shown by screening procedures. *(Fig. 74)*

Not infrequently in Cushing's syndrome, signs and symptoms of excess androgenicity occur. These may lead to precocious puberty in the prepubertal boy and to hirsutism or even virilism in the female. In the adult male, of course, no obvious androgenic effect is observed. These androgenic effects are not seen from pure glucocorticoid induced Cushing's syndrome (medicamentosa), but are due to the effect of excess adrenal androgens produced directly or more often by their conversion to testosterone in peripheral tissue. Such androgenic signs of this nature are much more frequent in adrenal tumor Cushing's syndrome than with pituitary Cushing's syndrome.

74

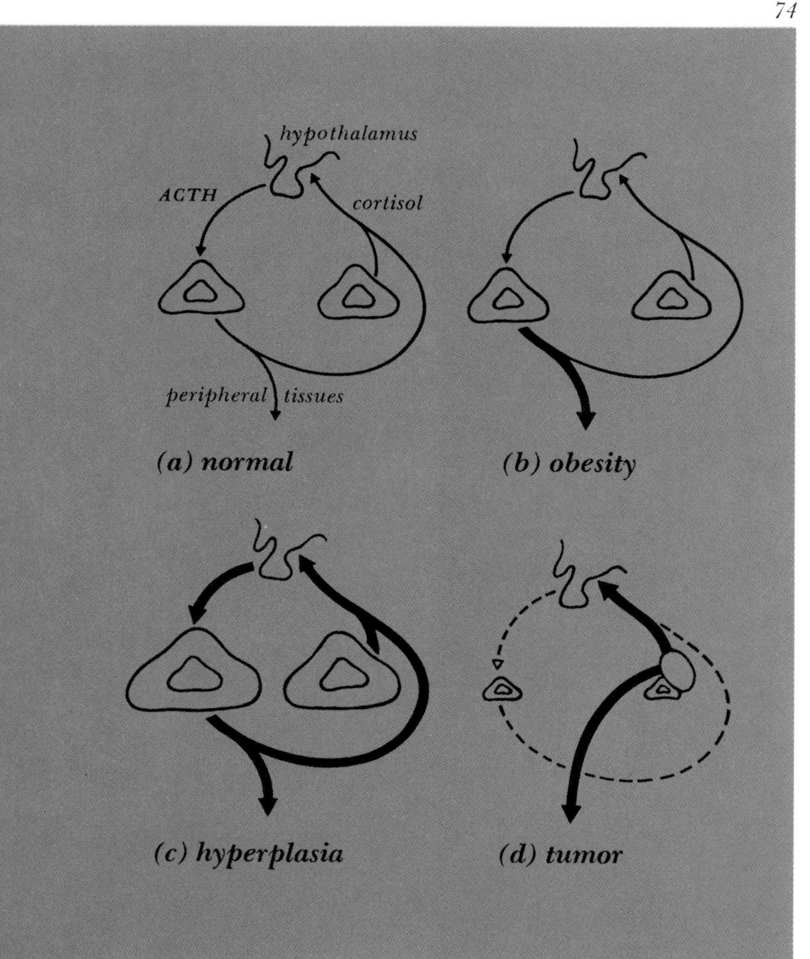

Diagnosis

The presence of even one of the more frequent signs or symptoms of Cushing's syndrome in a young female should suggest hypercortisolism as a possible cause. If, in addition, routine laboratory findings suggest a relatively low lymphocyte count with mild neutrophilia or mild polycythemia, an abnormal post-cibum blood glucose concentration or hypokalemic alkalosis, further diagnostic steps should be taken.

The diagnosis of Cushing's syndrome is a two-step process: 1. The presence of Cushing's syndrome is established; 2. The cause of the Cushing's syndrome is then determined.

Screening Tests for Cushing's Syndrome

Twenty-four hour urine 17-OHCS or 17-KGS are too frequently normal in patients with mild Cushing's syndrome to be utilized for diagnostic aids. Although loss of diurnal variation in plasma cortisol is often present when urinary steroid metabolites are normal, Cushing's syndrome can exist with a normal diurnal variation. Moreover, the collection of morning and evening bloods to establish its presence or absence is awkward, time consuming and expensive, especially on an ambulatory outpatient basis.

The Overnight Dexamethasone Suppression Test: This is the simplest and most reliable screening test for Cushing's syndrome. 1 mg of dexamethasone is taken orally by the patient at 11 p.m. and the following morning a blood specimen for a plasma cortisol determination is obtained between 8 a.m. and 9 a.m. If this value is less than 4 μg per 100 ml, Cushing's syndrome is not present. If the value is greater than 20 μg per 100 ml, Cushing's syndrome is likely to be present. In hospitalized patients, or in those who are psychologically disturbed, or otherwise ill, values frequently fall between 5 and 20 μg per 100 ml. In these cases, the Two-Day Liddle Dexamethasone Suppression Test must be done before the diagnosis of Cushing's syndrome is presumed.

These tests are based on the knowledge that Cushing's syndrome is due either to a source of ACTH that cannot be as readily suppressed by glucocorticoids as normal ACTH, or to an autonomously secreting adrenal tumor. If both tests are abnormal and the steroid analyses are performed by a reliable laboratory, there is a greater than 95% chance that the patient has Cushing's syndrome. *(Fig. 75)*

The Two-Day Low Dose Suppression Test of Liddle: When results of the Overnight Dexamethasone Suppression Test are equivocal, this longer test should be used and can be performed by the patient at home. The patient must be carefully instructed how to collect twenty-four hour urine samples. 0.5 mg of dexamethasone is taken every six hours for two days and 17-OHCS or 17-KGS are determined on the twenty-four hour

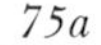

75a

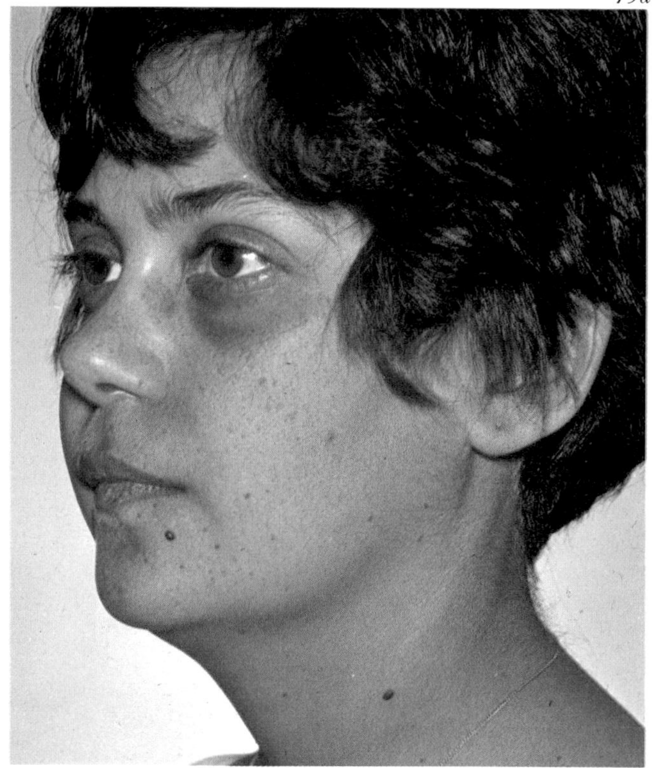

Fig. 74 *The abnormalities of control of cortisol secretion in obesity and Cushing's syndrome as compared to normal. In obesity there is enhanced peripheral utilization of cortisol leading to increased urinary steroid metabolites. Plasma* ACTH *and cortisol concentration remain normal, as does the feedback mechanism. In (c) the primary abnormality is in the set of the hypothalmus leading to an increased excretion of* ACTH, *cortisol and urinary metabolites. However, when the mechanism is interrupted as shown in Figure 72, the set is capable of responding but at a higher absolute glucocorticoid concentration. An autonomous tumor, either adenoma or carcinoma arising from the adrenal gland, such as in Figure 73, produces suppression of* ACTH *release from the pituitary leading to atrophy of the contralateral and ipsolateral adrenal cortex. Since the hypothalmus is completely suppressed, addition of dexamethasone to the plasma cannot produce further suppression and no decrease in urine steroid excretion occurs, Fig. 74d.*

Fig. 75a,b,c,d *Marked pigmentation in a young female with Cushing's syndrome which occurred six years following bilateral total adrenalectomy for bilateral hyperplasia (75a). Plasma* ACTH *levels were exceedingly high and were associated with an increase in the size of the pituitary fossa (75b & c). The pituitary tumor is usually a chromophobe adenoma and secretes both* ACTH *and* β MSH *in excess. The latter produces pigmentation (75d). This is compared to a normal hand. This condition was first described by Dr. D.H. Nelson and has been called Nelson's syndrome.*

75b

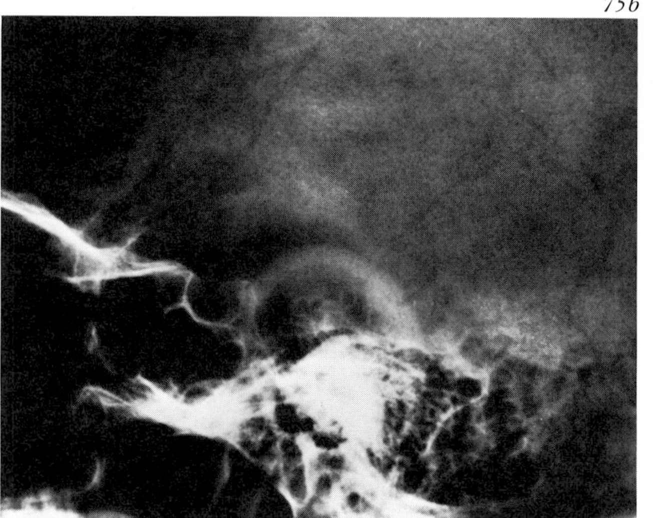

75c

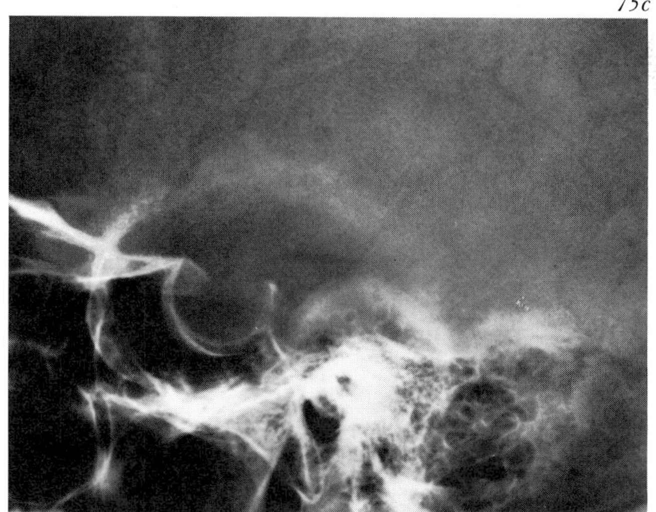

75d

Fig. 76 *Pre- and post-operative facial features of a patient with Cushing's syndrome due to adrenal adenoma.*

Fig. 77 *Reproduction of an x-ray of the skull of this patient (Fig. 76), showing the marked demineralization of the clinoid processes. Osteoporosis of this severity is rarely seen except in Cushing's syndrome.*

Fig. 78 *Marked osteoporosis of the lumbar spine of this patient (Fig. 76), with an adrenal adenoma. Bone substance has been lost and vertebral bodies have collapsed.*

Fig. 79 *Plasma cortisol and urinary 17-hydroxysteroids in a patient with Cushing's syndrome due to adrenal hyperplasia. Note the marked fluctuation in plasma cortisol concentration and the urinary steroid suppression to less than 50% of control on the "large dose" dexamethasone suppression test. With metyrapone (M) ingestion, there is a distinct rise in plasma and urinary cortisol in response to the released* ACTH. *Adrenal venous blood cortisol levels obtained by the catheter on the last day were equal in both the right (276 µg %) and left (262 µg %) adrenal veins. The vena cava concentration was 24 µg %.*

Fig. 80a & b *Adrenal venogram (PA) showing the enlarged adrenal glands in this patient (Fig. 79). The vascular pattern is "spread-out," especially on the right.*

76

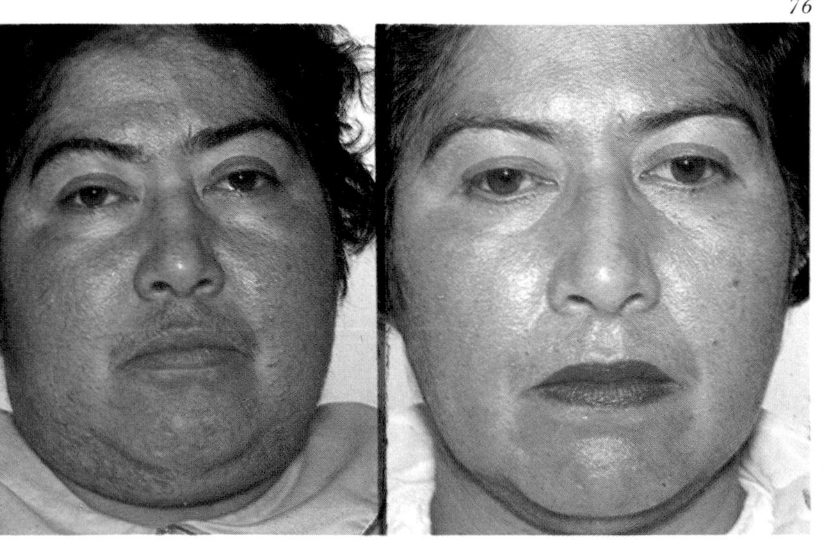

77

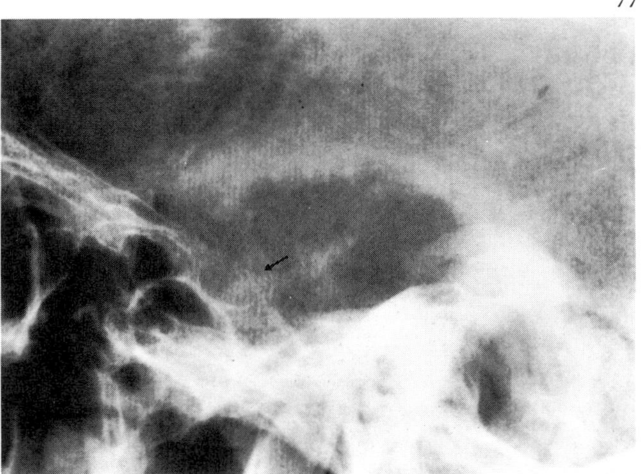

urines collected during the time of ingestion of the drug. Normal subjects will show on the second day a 17-OHCS excretion rate of less than 3.5 mg per twenty-four hours, or 17-KGS of less than 5 mg per twenty-four hours (over 95% of normal subjects). If the values are done in a reliable laboratory and are greater than this, the patient should be admitted to hospital for a more exacting diagnostic investigation.

Differential Diagnosis of Cushing's Syndrome

If the above two screening tests are abnormal, it is virtually certain the patient has hypercortisolism. It then remains to establish the etiology. This currently requires hospitalization. Twenty-four hour urine samples are collected continuously and the standard Dexamethasone Suppression Test of Liddle is carried out. *(Fig. 76-78)* On day one and two, routine blood chemistries, chest X-rays and physical examinations are done. All medications should be stopped prior to hospitalization. Control urinary steroids are collected on day one and two. On day three and four, 0.5 mg of dexamethasone is given to the patient every six hours and on day five and six this is increased to 2 mg of dexamethasone every six hours. Day seven is a control day; on day eight an adrenal venogram is done. Samples for plasma cortisol are taken from the right and left adrenal vein and from the superior and inferior vena cava.

Interpretation—*Adrenal Hyperplasia:* Less than 50% suppression of urinary cortisol metabolites from the two day control average on the low dose dexamethasone and a greater than 50% suppression on the second day of the high dose indicates adrenal hyperplasia. *(Fig. 79)*

Venogram: A normal or slightly increased size of both adrenals in the venogram may be seen. The plasma cortisol concentration from both the right and left adrenal vein are nearly equal and much higher than the superior vena cava sample. *(Fig. 80 a & b)*

Adrenal Tumor: 1. No suppression of urinary cortisol is observed at either dose of dexamethasone. *(Fig. 81)* 2. The venogram outlines a tumor in the left or right adrenal. Cortisol concentration is high on the side of the tumor and equal to that of the superior vena cava from the adrenal vein on the contralateral suppressed adrenal gland. *(Figs. 82-83)*

In the future it is likely these cumbersome diagnostic methods will be supplanted by simpler techniques, using simultaneously determined plasma ACTH and cortisol. If the ACTH concentration is high in the presence of relatively high concentration of cortisol, when the Overnight Suppression Test is done, Cushing's syndrome is likely to be present and due to ACTH excess. If ACTH is absent in the presence of a high cortisol, an adrenal tumor would be present. Adrenal venography could then be immediately performed to firmly establish the adrenal pathology, this is particularly impor-

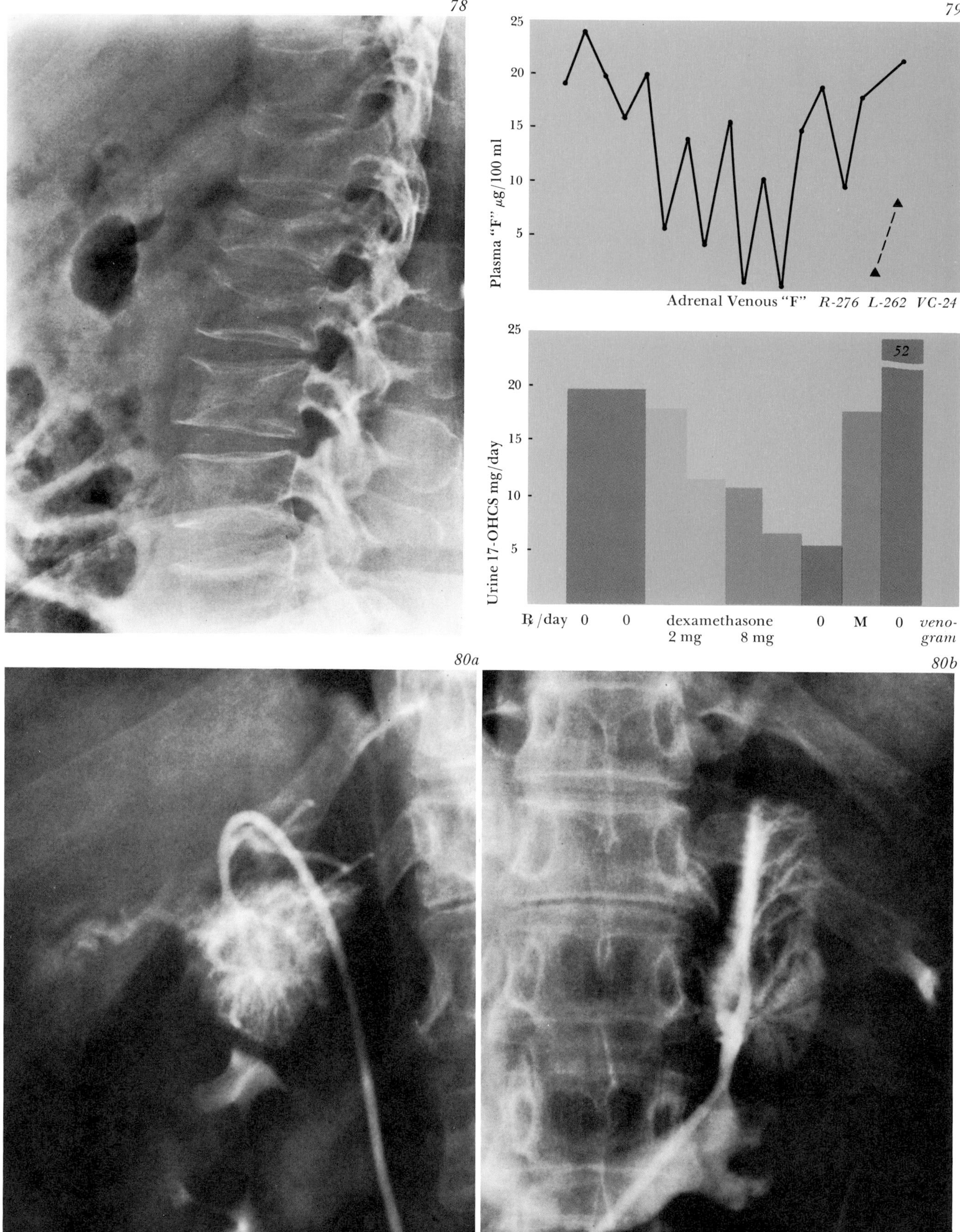
78
79
25
20
15
10
5
Plasma "F" µg/100 ml
Adrenal Venous "F" R-276 L-262 VC-24
25
20
15
10
5
52
Urine 17-OHCS mg/day
℞/day 0 0 dexamethasone 0 M 0 veno-
2 mg 8 mg gram
80a
80b

Fig. 81 *Clinical "work-up" on a patient with an adrenal adenoma. Note the lack of variation in plasma cortisol and the lack of cortisol suppression even during the time of large dose dexamethasone treatment. Metyrapone (M) leads to a fall in plasma and urinary cortisol. The adrenal venous blood cortisol concentration from the right adrenal gland (100 µg %) is much higher than from the left (21 µg %). The latter is equivalent to that of the peripheral plasma because of suppression of adrenal cortical secretion in the left adrenal. The concentration in the vena cava was 12 µg %.*

Fig. 82 *Adrenal venogram of this patient showing the tumor in the right gland.*

Fig. 83 *Cross-section of the adenoma from this patient (Fig. 81) showing the marked involution of the adrenal gland attached to this adenoma.*

Fig. 84 *Alterations in various tests of adrenal function in normal patients, patients with obesity, patients with anxiety, patients receiving estrogens and in three cases of Cushing's syndrome.*

81

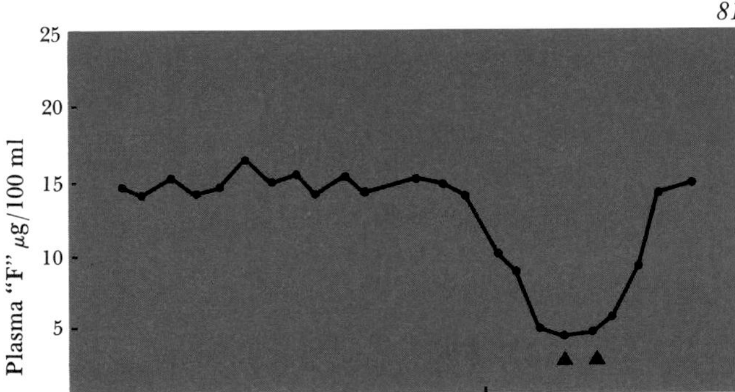

Adrenal Venous "F" *R-100 L-21 VC-12*

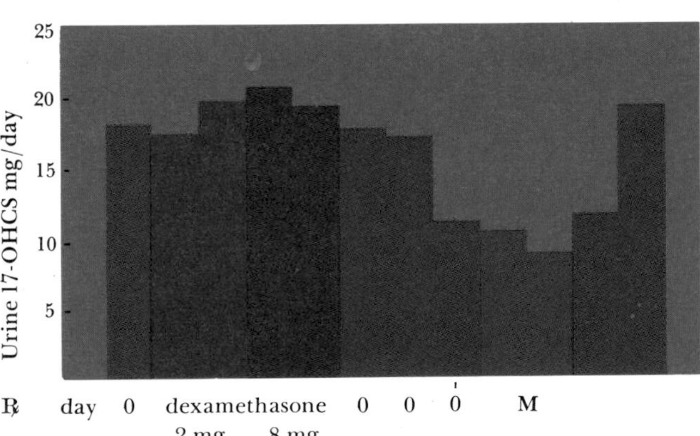

℞ day 0 dexamethasone 0 0 0 M
2 mg 8 mg

82

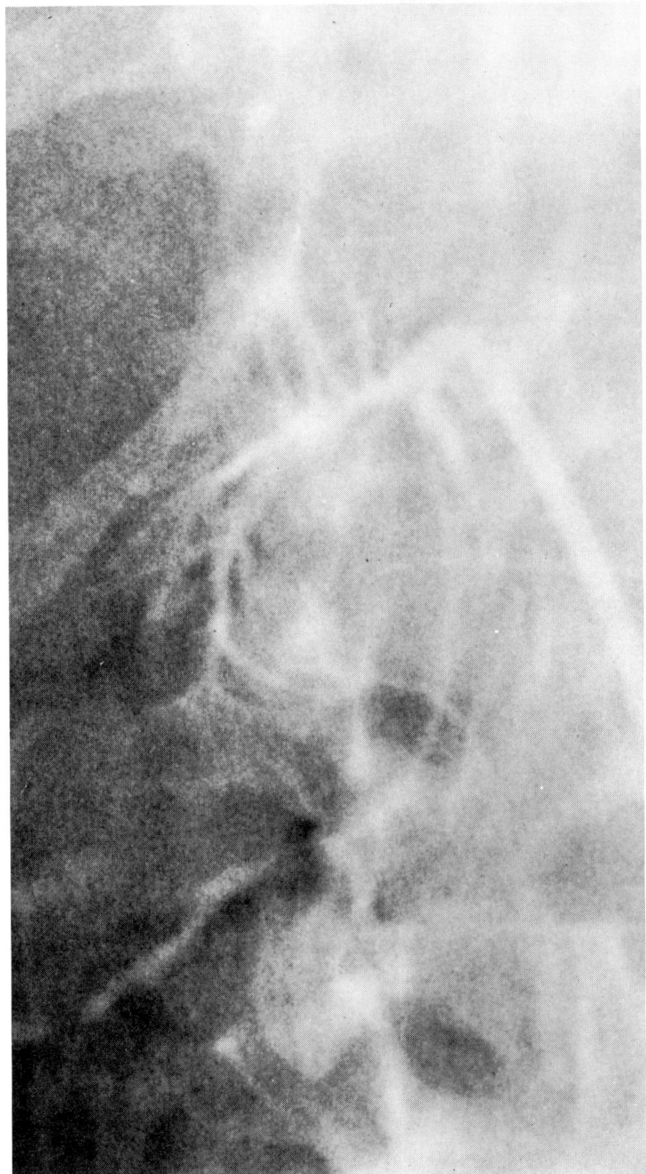

83

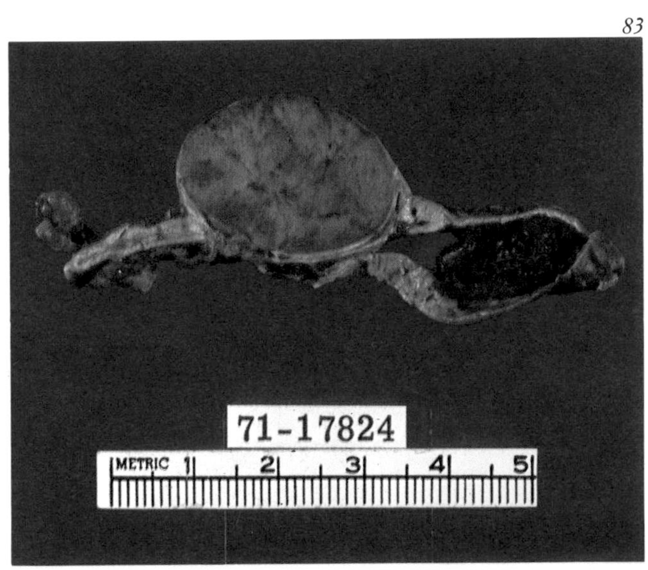

tant if surgical treatment is contemplated. There is a distinct possibility that the non-endocrine tumors produce ACTH which can be shown to be immunologically or chemically different from normal pituitary ACTH. Possibly, in the not too distant future, this will facilitate differentiation of the ectopic from the pituitary excess ACTH causes of Cushing's syndrome.

Obesity: An increased cortisol secretion rate is found in approximately one-third of patients with obesity. It is due to an increased catabolism of cortisol in peripheral tissues and is not associated with an increase in plasma cortisol concentration. Diurnal variation is present and normal suppressibility is found. Urine steroid secretion rates may be as high as twice normal due to the excess metabolism. There is a good correlation of body surface area with the increased cortisol secretion rate. This rate will return to normal when normal lean body mass is attained by dieting. Since obesity may be associated with mild hirsutism, weakness and oligomenorrhea, it is the commonest diagnostic problem encountered in the differential diagnosis of Cushing's syndrome. It is ruled out by suppression testing. *(Fig. 84)*

Estrogens: Even the small amount of estrogenic substances contained in birth control pills may increase the production of CBG by the liver. This will give rise to an elevated plasma cortisol concentration, but since free cortisol is near normal, urine cortisol metabolism and suppressibility are normal. Although the Dexamethasone Overnight Suppression Test will usually give a normal result, it is best for the patient to discontinue these drugs for at least two weeks before the test is carried out.

Treatment

The treatment of Cushing's syndrome depends on the diagnosis.

Pituitary excess ACTH syndrome. If the patient has mild Cushing's syndrome, without severe osteoporosis, psychologic problems or hypertension, it is usually best to attempt pituitary irradiation with up to 5,000 rads. This will result in a cure in six to twelve months in 50% of the patients. High voltage proton beam therapy may give even better results.

Bilateral total adrenalectomy. If Cushing's disease is severe, or if there has been failure of pituitary irradiation, bilateral total adrenalectomy is the only certain cure for Cushing's syndrome. However, it cannot be looked upon as recommended treatment, for the physician is simply substituting a more curable form of disease for a lethal disease. The patient's Addison's disease will now need to be treated for the rest of his life.

Medical treatment with anti-cortisol drugs has been attempted on an experimental basis, but it is not currently recommended.

If an adrenal tumor is present, exploratory surgery and removal of an adrenal adenoma is curative. If carcinoma is found, the primary tumor is usually removed and adrenolytic drugs are utilized for treatment of the metastases. The tumor is usually quite malignant and death within five years is common.

84

Test Alterations	*normal*	*obesity*	*anxiety*	*estrogen treatment*	*adrenal hyperplasia*	*adrenal adenoma*	*adrenal carcinoma*
8:00 AM Plasma Cortisol	N	N	N or ↑	↑	↑ N	↑ N	↑
Single Dose Dexamethasone Suppression Test	↓	↓	→	↓→	→	→	→
Control Urine 17-KGS, 17-OHCS	N	↑	N	N	↑ N	↑ N	↑
Small Dose 2 Day Dexamethasone Suppression Test	↓	↓	↓	↓	→	→	→
Large Dose 2 Day Dexamethasone Suppression Test	↓	↓	↓	↓	↓	→	→
Metyrapone Test	↑	↑	↑	↑	↑↑	→↓	→↓

7 Conn's Syndrome

Primary Hyperaldosteronism: Primary hyperaldosteronism is important because it is a curable cause of hypertension. It accounts for approximately 1% of patients with hypertension. Other curable causes of increased blood pressure are: coarctation of the aorta; unilateral renal disease; pheochromocytoma; Cushing's syndrome; certain types of the adrenal genital syndrome.

Primary hyperaldosteronism is due to a single adrenocortical adenoma in approximately 80% of cases. *(Fig. 85)* It occurs twice as frequently in females as males and is usually found between the ages of thirty and fifty. Bilateral hyperplasia is found more frequently in children, and when in adults, is usually found as bilateral adenomatous hyperplasia (15%). Carcinoma is rare.

A patient with Conn's syndrome usually presents to the physician with hypertension. Hypokalemia is usually present. The hypertension is characteristically mild and may be associated with headache. All clinical findings may be attributed to prolonged mineralocorticoid excess by an autonomously secreting tumor. This suppresses the renin angiotensin system and characteristically the high aldosterone secretion rate is associated with very low plasma renin concentrations. Such a condition is in contrast to the hyperaldosteronism associated with edema as in nephrosis, congestive heart failure and cirrhotic ascites where the elevated aldosterone sometimes found, is secondary to renal stimulation of renin and is therefore called secondary hyperaldosteronism. (In these cases the renin aldosterone system is responsive to volume expanding maneuvers and provides a basis for the separation of primary from secondary hyperaldosteronism.)

The excess aldosterone of primary aldosteronism leads to sodium retention and potassium loss. Plasma volume expands until the escape mechanism occurs. The expanded volume probably produces the hypertension but the mechanism of hypertension in hyperaldosteronism is by no means clear. Secondary hyperaldosteronism does not produce hypertension. Although escape from the sodium retaining effect of aldosterone occurs within a few days, the potassium losing effect is not lost. Hypokalemia is characteristic and may be so severe as to give rise to weakness and muscle paralysis. This weakness is more prominent in the extremities than in the facial muscles. The low potassium level may even lead to tetany, paresthesias and electrocardiographic changes. Long continued hypokalemia produces vasopressin resistant polyuria due to alterations in water transport in the distal tubule of the nephron (kalipenic nephropathy). Polydipsia may occasionally result from this. The hypokalemia may lead to a mild alkalosis with mild bicarbonate excess in the plasma. Carbohydrate intolerance may occasionally result from the prolonged hypokalemia. In spite of the low potassium, the stimulating effect of aldosterone on distal tubular potassium secretion usually produces a relatively high urine content of potassium (greater than 40 meq/day). This is of some diagnostic value.

Diagnosis: Primary hyperaldosteronism is usually only suspected in the patient with hypertension who has repeated unprovoked hypokalemia. (Potassium less than 3.5 meq/liter.) The most common cause of hypokalemia in hypertension is thiazide diuretic treatment. At least three serum potassium determinations at intervals of a few days should be obtained before thiazide diuretics are used to treat hypertension. Although it has been suggested that normokalemic hyperaldosteronism might be a common cause of hypertension, this has proven to be distinctly unusual, and a careful physician can be satisfied that repeated normal potassium determinations in his hypertensive patients rule out primary aldosteronism. Malignant hypertension frequently is associated with elevated aldosterone secretion rates and hypokalemia. This is almost never due to a primary tumor with elevated plasma renin concentration. This is a type of secondary aldosteronism and responds to volume expansion by reductions of renin and aldosterone secretions.

If repeated serum potassium determinations in a patient receiving a liberal sodium intake are below 3.5 meq/liter, Conn's syndrome should be suspected. Since urinary aldosterone methods measure only a small fraction of the aldosterone secreted, much greater reliance is now placed on serum aldosterone determinations by radioimmunoassay. Because aldosterone secretion is autonomous and excessive, the renin angiotensin system is suppressed. In normal subjects and in secondary aldosteronism, it is possible to suppress plasma aldosterone concentration to low levels by volume expansion. The patient is given dietary salt as 2 grams of sodium chloride four times a day which, together with his normal intake, will insure a sodium intake of approximately 200 meq/day. He is then given a potent mineralocorticoid fludrocortisone, 0.2 mg t.i.d. for three days. On the morning of the third day, blood for plasma aldosterone is obtained, and if the value is below 5 μg/100 ml, primary aldosterone is not present. If it is greater than 10 μg/100 ml and, in addition, plasma renin is low (less than 300 units), primary aldosterone is probably present. The patient should then be admitted to a hospital for adrenal venography. Plasma aldosterone will usually be high in the adrenal vein from the adrenal gland containing the lesion and in about 70% of cases a tumor is seen on the retrograde venogram. Since plasma renin is low in at least 25% of patients with essential hypertension, much less creditability is placed on this measurement as the assay is complicated and unreliable. However, it does give additional information, for, in the face of continued excessive aldosterone secretion, renin levels are usually low and do not normally increase with the assumption of the upright posture for four hours.

Treatment: The patient with Conn's syndrome should usually be treated for at least a month with high doses of an aldosterone antagonist (spironolactone—400 mg/day) to correct the hypokalemia, improve the hypertension and lessen the risks of surgery for the patient. This is also an excellent therapeutic trial to supplement the previously obtained information as well as providing the physician a prognosis on the outcome of surgery. If blood pressure is reduced to normal levels, a good response from surgery is probable. In some older patients, surgery may be postponed indefinitely if this medical treatment is satisfactory.

Adrenal venography has greatly simplified the surgeon's task in management of Conn's syndrome. *(Fig.*

Fig. 85 *Photograph of a typical adrenal adenoma producing Conn's syndrome.*

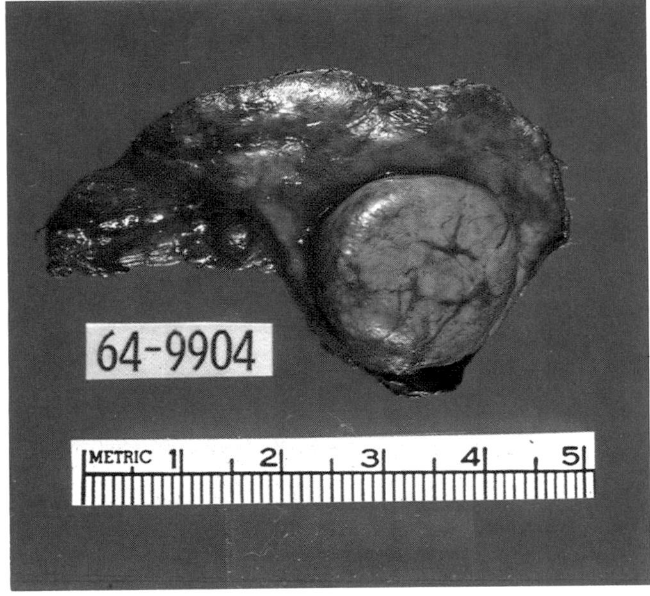

86

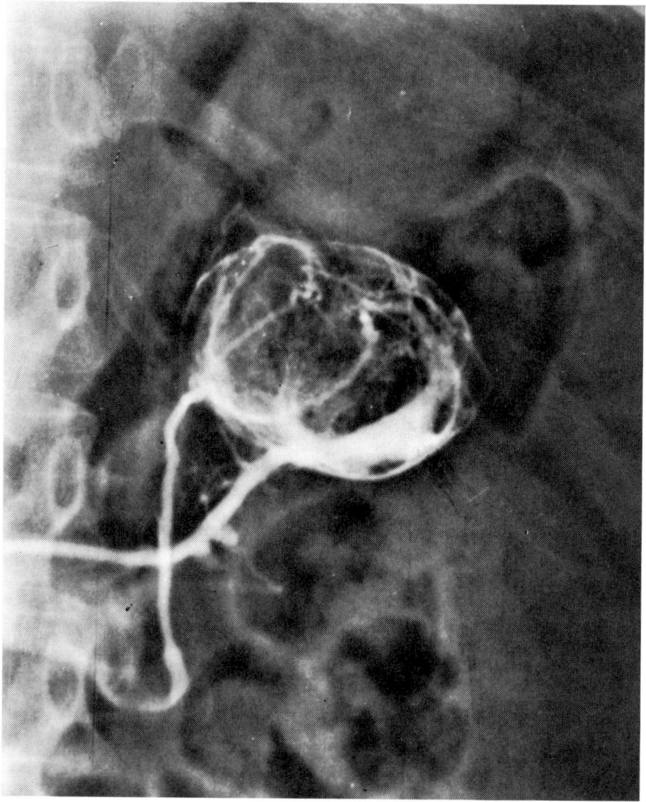

87

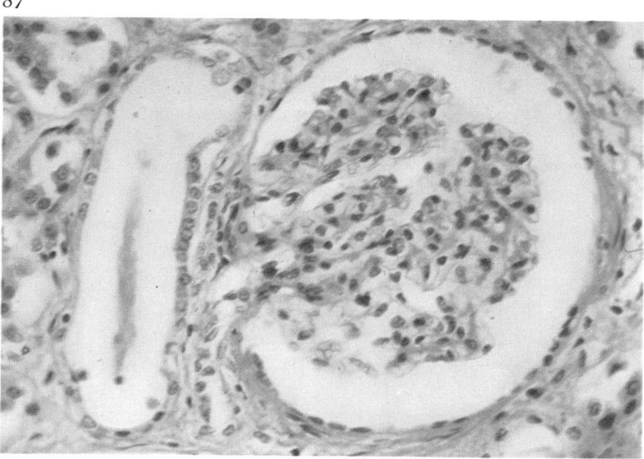

88

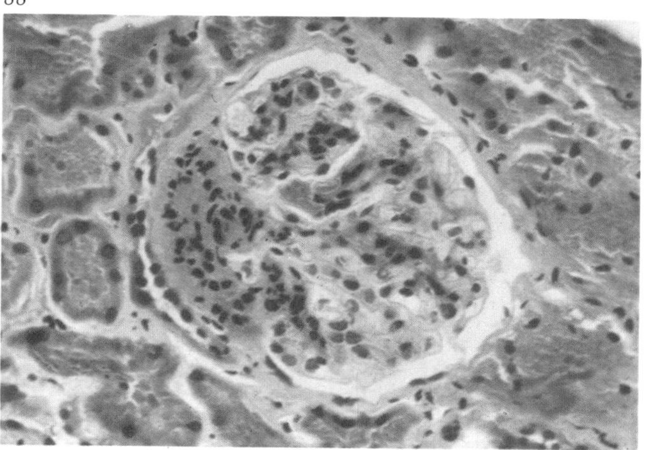

86) The adenoma often is small and may escape visual detection. In the past, without an adrenal venograph, the surgeon had to expose and carefully palpate both glands to be certain an adenoma or that bilateral adenomas were not present. Adrenal venography with adrenal effluent aldosterone determinations precisely informs the surgeon which gland or glands are at fault, so exposure of both glands is unnecessary unless the results indicate bilateral disease.

Usually, but not always, the hypertension is cured by surgery unless bilateral hyperplasia is present. As in hypertension from any cause, cardiovascular, cerebrovascular and renal destructive lesions may have become irreversibly progressive by the time the adrenal tumor is removed.

Other Causes of Hyperaldosteronism

Secondary hyperaldosterone. The normal response of the renin angiotensin system to volume depletion is to increase aldosterone secretion leading to sodium and water retention to restore the plasma volume towards normal. Thus, sodium deficiency, blood loss, renal artery constriction, sequestration of blood on the venous side of the circulation, ascites and any cause of decreased renal blood flow and pressure lead to increased aldosterone secretion. In these cases renin is elevated and the system responds normally to blood volume expansion by saline infusion or with mineralocorticoid ingestion.

Bartter's Syndrome

A rare, but important syndrome was described by Dr. Bartter in 1962. In these patients high secretion rates of aldosterone are associated with moderate to severe hypokalemia with extremely high plasma renin concentration, but for unknown reasons do not have hypertension and edema. The high plasma concentration of renin found in this syndrome seems to be due to marked juxtaglomerular apparatus hyperplasia usually found on renal biopsy. *(Figs. 87, 88)* It has been postulated that this juxtaglomerular hyperplasia is due to an intrinsic renal lesion so that high concentrations of sodium leak directly from the glomerulus to the macula densa and lead to sustained over-secretion of renin. It has also been suggested to be due to decreased sensitivity of the vascular bed to angiotensin with a resultant high renin concentration.

Fig. 86 *Adrenal venogram of a large adenoma producing Conn's syndrome.*

Fig. 87 *Cross-section of a normal glomerulus showing the small juxtamedullary body in association with the macula densa (x100) H & E.*

Fig. 88 *Marked hyperplasia of the juxtaglomerular body in a patient with Bartter's syndrome (x100) H & E.*

8 Congenital Adrenal Hyperplasia

Adrenal Biosynthetic Disorders: The most common adrenal disorder encountered in pediatric practice is the Adrenogenital syndrome. This form of congenital adrenal hyperplasia is due to an enzymatic block resulting in deficient hydroxylation at the C-21 position of the steroid molecule. There have been to date a total of five such blocks described in the steroid synthetic pathway and there is every likelihood that an enzyme deficient syndrome to fit each enzyme in the pathway will eventually be described. *(Figs. 89, 90)*

There are usually two immediate consequences of such a block: 1. The steroid intermediates directly behind the block build up in the adrenal and spill out into the blood; 2. There may be a deficiency of steroids normally produced beyond the block.

Since the last and most important of these steroids in the pathway is cortisol, ACTH is produced in excess in an attempt to overcome the effect of glucocorticoid deficiency by restoring plasma cortisol to near normal levels. This leads to adrenal hyperplasia and often to a huge excess of adrenal steroid intermediates flooding the body. Normally they are found in the peripheral circulation only in trace quantities. These intermediate steroids may then directly produce biologic effects or be altered in non-adrenal tissues to other biologically active steroids. The characteristics of all enzymatic defects are: 1. A varying degree of cortisol deficiency; 2. Adrenal hyperplasia; and 3. Various clinical manifestations due to the excess preblock intermediates formed.

21-Hydroxylase Deficiency: This, the most common defect is due to autosomal recessive inheritance and is observed much more frequently in girls than boys. The incidence is controversial, being reported as often as 1/5,000 births in one series and as infrequently as 1/67,000 births in another series. *(Figs. 89-94)*

The result of a C-21 hydroxylase block is to inhibit both the glucocorticoid and mineralocorticoid pathway. The ACTH excess due to the cortisol deficiency pushes the steroid synthetic pathway prior to pregnenolone formation leading to an excess of the precursors 17-hydroxypregnenolone, 17-hydroxyprogesterone and progesterone, which are then shunted toward the androgen pathway. The excess androstenedione secreted is

Fig. 89 *Enlarged clitoris in an eight-month-old baby girl. Urinary 17-ketosteroids were twice normal, pregnanetriol was twice normal, and plasma testosterone level was 377 nanograms/100 ml, almost four times normal. Figures 89, 90, 91, and 94 are congenital adrenal hyperplasia due to a 21-hydroxylase deficiency in a brother and sister. (See Fig. 90)*

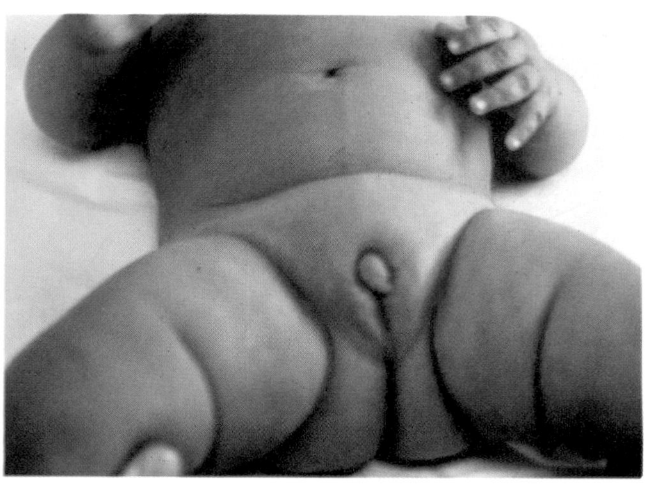

90

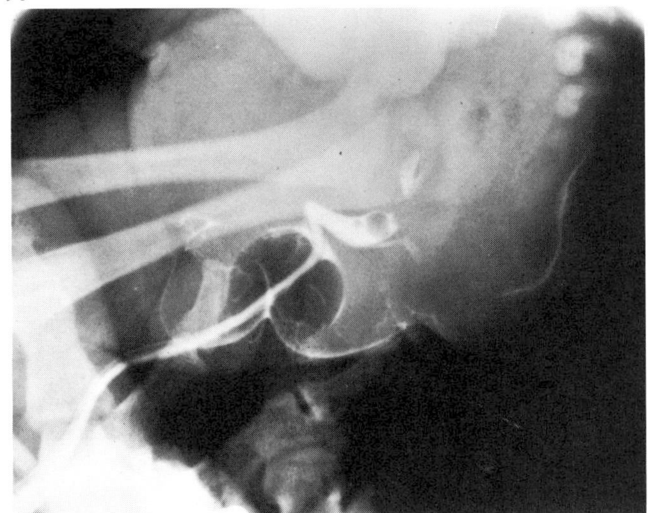

91

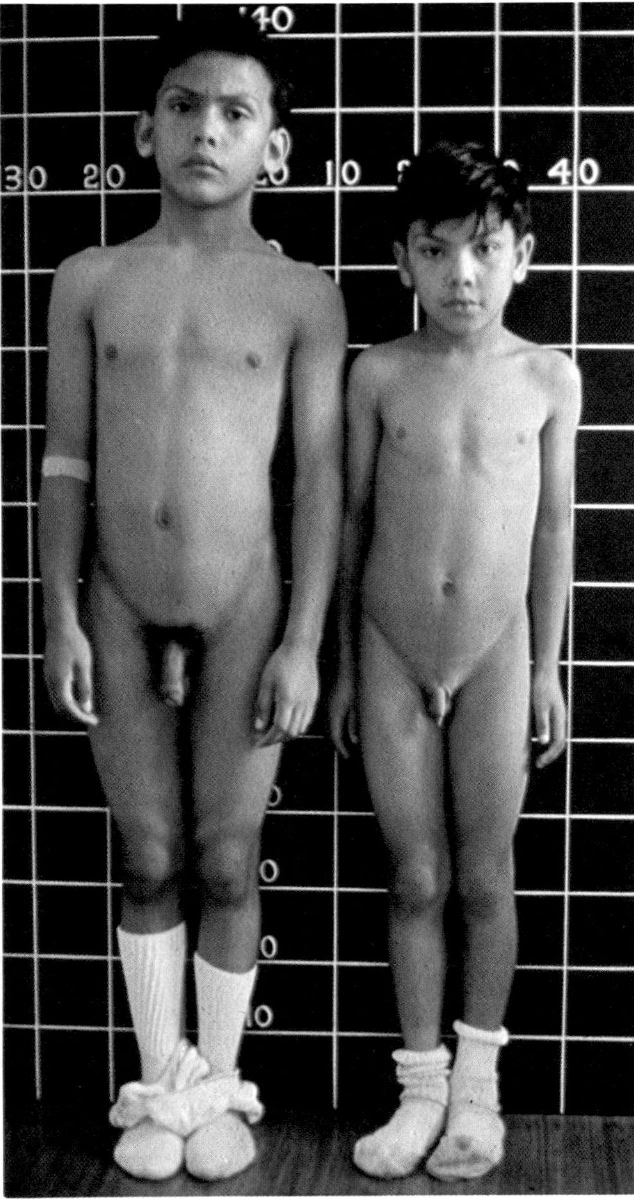

then converted by peripheral tissues to testosterone. The latter leads to virilization of the external genitalia. In utero and at birth, varying degrees of virilization in the female are found. The excess 17-hydroxyprogesterone and progesterone are metabolized in the liver and excreted in the urine as pregnanetriol and pregnandiol. Excess excretion of these in the infant are used to confirm the presence of this defect. The increased dehydroepiandrosterone (DHEA) and androstenedione gives rise to large quantities of urinary 17-keto steroids.

The defect may vary in its completeness. If severe, the mineralocorticoid pathway may be so inhibited that salt wasting occurs and the infant will die of dehydration if untreated. In its mildest form, the androgenic effects only may be manifest at puberty, e.g., hirsutism, poor breast development and amenorrhoea.

Usually the defect is intermediate in severity. A female infant is born with a large clitoris and if untreated she will grow rapidly with a masculine habitus. Pubic hair will appear early, a deep voice may appear some years later and at puberty menarche does not occur. It must be emphasized that most of the biological androgenicity in this syndrome derives from the testosterone produced in non-adrenal tissues by the conversion of the precursors DHEA and androstenedione to testosterone. There is a negligible direct androgenic effect from the excess DHEA and androsterone, very unimportant androgens in the human. *(Fig. 95)* The simplest test, therefore, for following adequate replacement treatment is to measure serum testosterone levels and replace the cortisol until testosterone is maintained in the normal range.

Other Enzymatic Defects

Desmolase Deficiency: Since no steroid hormones can be produced in this defect, it is incompatible with life. At autopsy, the infants have been found to have large fat-laden adrenals.

3B-hydroxydehydrogenase defect: This defect is also incompatible with prolonged life and no affected infants have survived more than a few months. Behind

Fig. 90 *Instillation of contrast material into the vagina of this patient (Fig. 89) revealed a normal infantile vagina, uterus and fallopian tubes.*

Fig. 91 *The patient on left is the six-year-three-month-old brother of the patient in Figure 89 (his height age is 13 years). Urinary 17-ketosteroids were 28 mg per 24 hours, pregnanetriol was 50 mg per 24 hours, and plasma testosterone was 472 nanograms/100 ml. This is almost five times normal. Secondary sex characteristics are well advanced. He has facial hair, and a deep voice, which had been present since the age of two years. A diagnosis of adrenal genital syndrome was made following diagnosis in his sister, shortly after her birth. Shown on the right is a normal brother at age eight years.*

Fig. 92 *The five adrenal biosynthetic disorders described due to deficiency of major enzyme systems.*

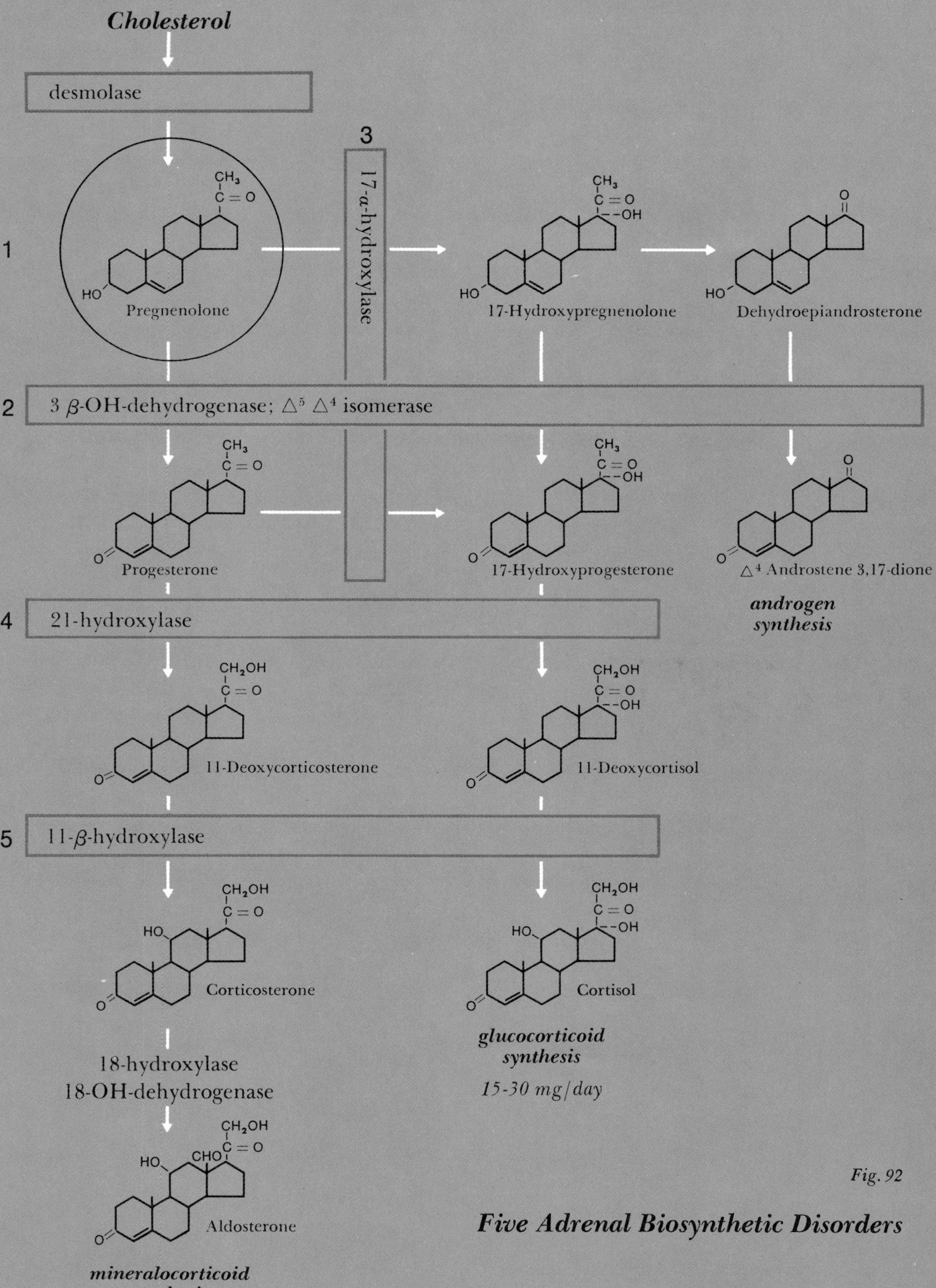

Fig. 92

Five Adrenal Biosynthetic Disorders

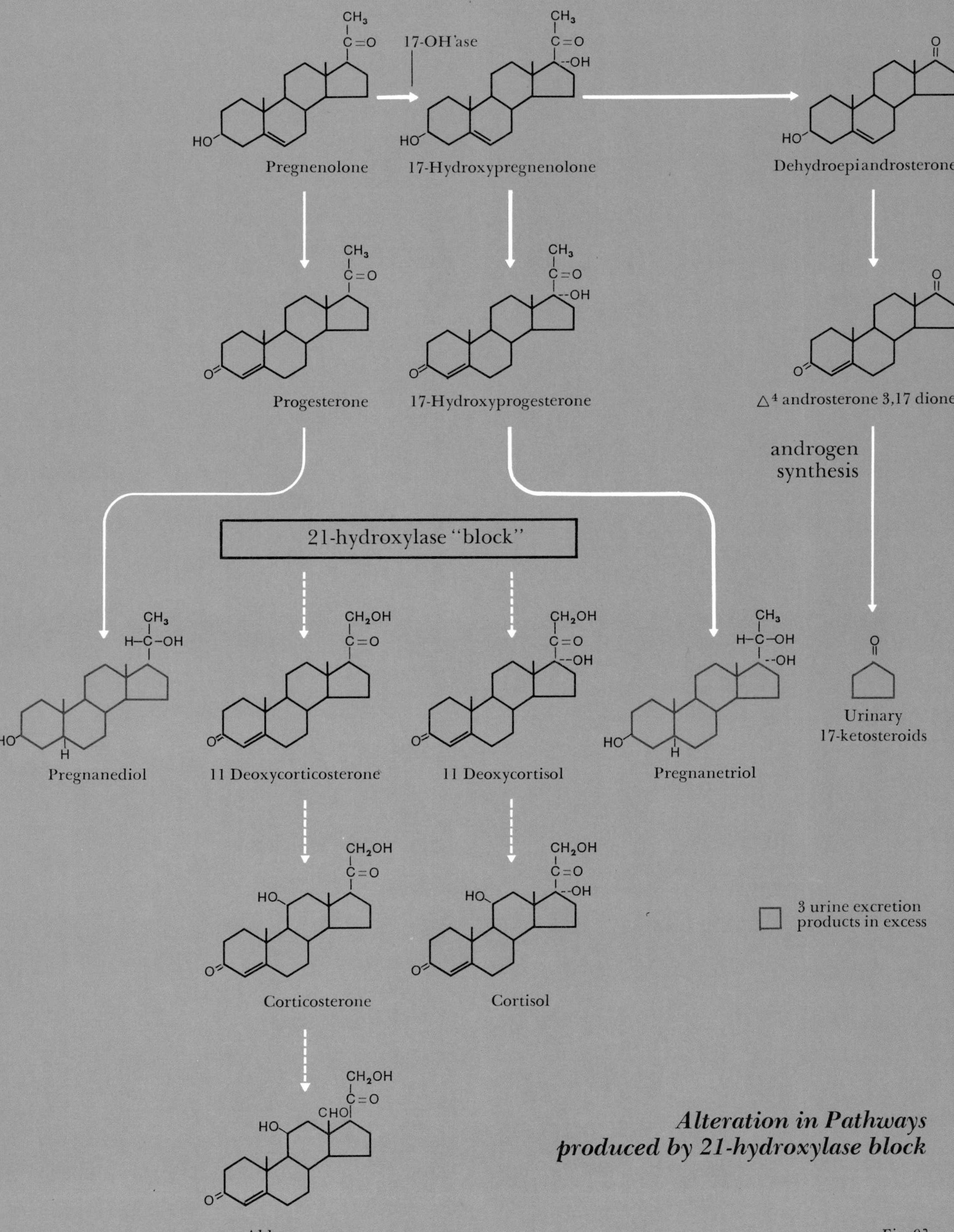

Alteration in Pathways produced by 21-hydroxylase block

Fig. 93

94a

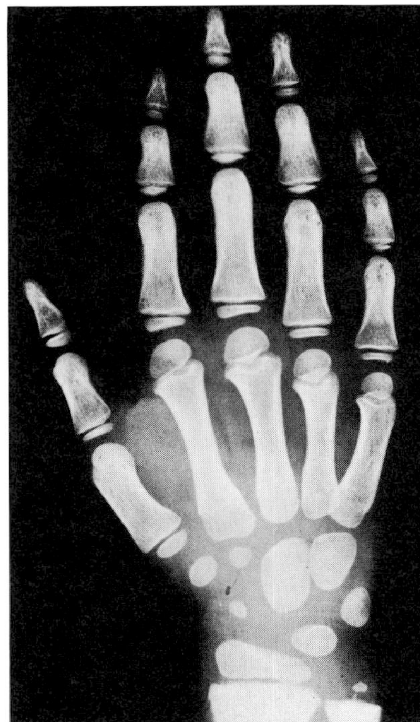

94b

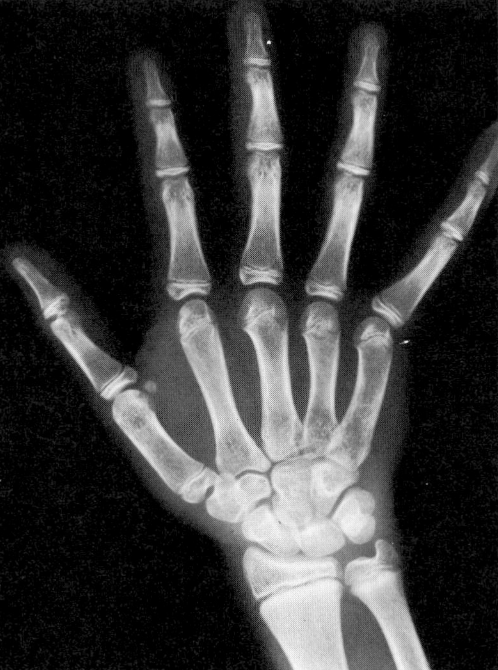

94c

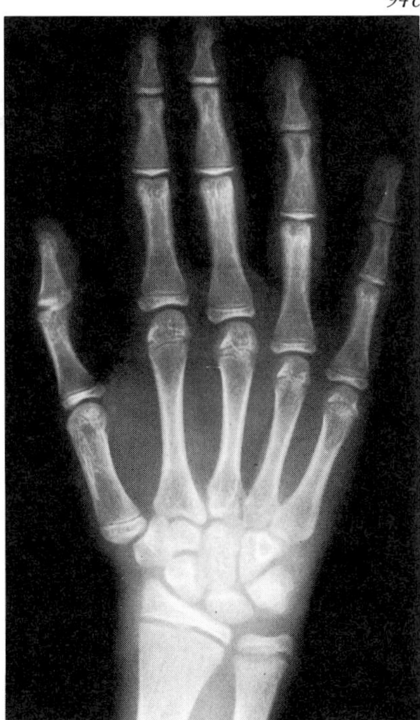

the block—pregnenolone accumulates and is shunted on to the production of DHEA, thus leading to excess androsterone production. In the liver and other peripheral tissues, androsterone is converted to testosterone which gives rise to androgenicity. Girls are therefore born with mild virilism and boys with hypospadias.

C-17 Hydroxylase Deficiency: This defect is compatible with life, for C-17 hydroxy steroids can be effectively replaced by a weaker C-11 glucocorticoid precursor, corticosterone. In animals such as the rabbit and rat, this is the only glucocorticoid manufactured. In this syndrome, corticosteroid secretion is excessive and controls the excess ACTH secretion relatively well. However, its immediate precursor 11-deoxycorticosterone, a very active mineralocorticoid, is also produced in excess, and therefore, a hyperaldosterone-like syndrome develops. Since, the C-17 defect is present in the ovaries and testes, a deficiency of both male and female hormones occur and both sexes are of the female phenotype, regardless of genetic sex.

C-21 Hydroxylase Deficiency: Previously discussed, page 61

C-11 Hydroxylase Deficiency: The 11-hydroxy group is necessary for all biologically active corticosteroids and this defect results in a decrease of cortisol, corticosterone and aldosterone. This leads to a syndrome similar to the C-21 hydroxylase defect except that the potent mineralocorticoid, deoxycorticosterone is formed in excess and produces, in addition to virilization, a hyperaldosteronism-like picture. This syndrome presents early virilization with hypertension and hypokademia. This is a defect analagous to that observed by the administration of metyrapone to a normal subject.

Fig. 93 *Alterations in the pathways produced by the most common form of adrenal genital syndrome, 21-hydroxylase block. There is an increase in the urine of three excretion products, pregnanetriol, pregnanediol and urinary 17-ketosteroids.*

Fig. 94a,b,c *X-ray of the wrist of patient, Fig. 91, at the chronological age of six years and three months (Fig. 94b). Bone development is comparable to that of the hand from a normal thirteen-year-old boy (Fig. 94c). For contrast, the x-ray of a normal six-year-old boy is shown on the left (94a).*

Fig. 95 *Relative androgenicity ratios of androgens produced in man. Testosterone is arbitrarily assigned a ratio of 100.*

Relative Androgenicity *Fig. 95*

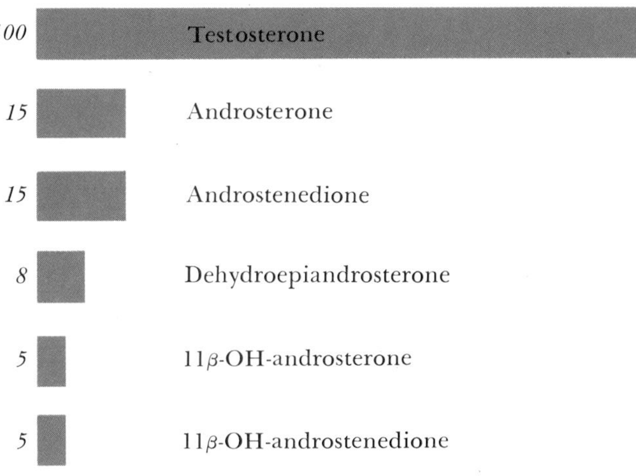

Glossary

Acidic Steroid—Any steroid such as the C_{18} estrogens with a phenolic A-ring. This renders the molecule a hydrogen donor in solution making it acidic.

ACTH (Adrenocorticotropin)—A 39 amino acid polypeptide produced in the pituitary gland which stimulates the secretion of adrenal steroids.

Addison's Disease—The syndrome first described by Thomas Addison resulting from destruction of the adrenal cortex. In modern terms, insufficiency of adrenal secretion of cortisol due to a variety of etiologies.

Adrenal Crisis—Shock due to acute adrenal insufficiency. This is mainly due to the absence of the adrenal glucocorticoid, cortisol.

Adrenal Androgen—Steroids produced by the adrenal cortex which are weakly androgenic or are converted by peripheral tissues to the potent androgen testosterone. They are the only androgens that have the C_{11} oxygen group and thus have been called the C_{11} androgens.

Aldosterone—The mineralocorticoid produced by the zona glomerulosa containing a C_{18} aldehyde group.

Androgens—Steroids which produce maleness.

Angiotensin—A pressor polypeptide produced in plasma that stimulates aldosterone secretion.

Bartter's Syndrome—A form of secondary aldosteronism caused by juxtaglomerular cell hyperplasia associated with extremely high levels of plasma renin.

Bound Steroids—Steroids bound to plasma protein by weak electrochemical forces.

CBG (Transcortin)—Corticosteroid binding globulin. α_2-globulin in plasma which specifically binds steroids containing the $\triangle^{4\text{-}3}$ ketone complex.

Competitive Protein Binding Cortisol—A method for measuring the steroid, cortisol, utilizing the competitive binding protein CBG. It is very sensitive and specific.

Conn's Syndrome—The syndrome described by Doctor Jerome Conn. It is due to the excessive excretion of aldosterone from an adrenal tumor or adrenal hyperplasia.

Conjugate Steroids—A form in which steroids are metabolized by a process occurring in the liver whereby steroids are conjugated with sulfates or glucuronates rendering them water soluble. They are biologically inactive and readily excretable through the kidneys.

Corticosteroids—This term includes the biologically active life-maintaining adrenocorticosteroids and their metabolites but excludes C_{19} steroids and progesterone. It is usually limited to the C_{21} steroids with three or more oxygen atoms.

Cortex—The outer zone of the adrenal gland; composed of the zona glomerulosa, zona fasciculata and zona reticularis.

Corticotrophin—See ACTH.

Corticotrophin Releasing Factor (CRF)—A small polypeptide produced in the median eminence which passes through the hypophyseal portal system and stimulates the secretion of ACTH from the pituitary.

Cortin—A term first applied to crude extracts of the adrenal gland containing many steroids.

Cortisol—The trivial name of the major glucocorticoid produced by the adrenal cortex, synonymous with hydrocortisone.

Cortisone—The trivial name of the first glucocorticoid utilized for the treatment of disease in man. It is synthesized but is produced in very minor amounts, if at all, in the normal human adrenal cortex.

Cortolone—A metabolite of tetrahydrocortisone produced in the liver by reduction of the 20-keto group to form a 20-hydroxyl radical. They are then conjugated with glucuronic acid and excreted in the urine.

Cortol—A metabolite of tetrahydrocortisol produced in the liver by reduction of the 20-keto group to form a 20-hydroxyl radical. They are then conjugated with glucuronic acid and excreted in the urine.

Cushing's Syndrome—A syndrome described by Dr. Harvey Cushing due to excessive secretion of adrenal steroids. It is now a term usually confined to the state due to secretion of glucocorticoids, although mineralocorticoid, androgenic and estrogenic effects are occasionally seen. The syndrome is most often produced by ingestion of synthetic glucocorticoids.

Desoxycorticosterone—The trivial name of the first adrenal steroid synthesized in 1937. It is primarily a mineralocorticoid but has very slight glucocorticoid effect.

DHEA (Dehydroepiandrosterone)—A steroid derived from the adrenal cortex is largely converted in the adrenal to $\triangle^4$ androstene 3, 17-dione which is then converted to androsterone and etiocholanolone. These are weakly androgenic substances which are measured in urine as 17-ketosteroids.

Estrogens—Substances which produce feminizing features. These are primarily produced by the ovary and are acidic C_{18} steroids.

Fetal Cortex—The large outer zone of the adrenal cortex present through embryonic life and persisting for a few days postpartum. This zone produces DHEA, which is utilized by the placenta for producing large amounts of estrogens necessary for the normal maintenance of pregnancy.

Fluorescent Cortisol—The term used for the method of measuring plasma cortisol by utilizing its fluorescent properties when mixed with an acidic solution.

Free Cortisol (Steroids)—The amount of cortisol (steroid) that is present in plasma or urine not bound or conjugated. It is thought to represent the biologically active steroid.

Glucocorticoids—Those steroids which predominately affect intermediary metabolism. They were originally named because of their glycogen storing effect on the liver.

Glucosiduronate—The conjugate of a steroid with glucuronic acid. This conjugation occurs in the liver and renders the steroid biologically inactive and water soluble.

Gluconeogenic Steroids—A term applied to glucocorticoids because the glycogenic effect is related to its stimulatory effect on gluconeogenesis.

Half-Life (T½)—The term applied to the biological half-life of steroids in plasma. It is the time required for the concentration of a steroid to fall by one-half its initial value with the understanding that no new glucocorticoid is added into the system.

Hirsutism—Excessive body hair in the female. It has occasionally been applied to males with excessive hair.

Hydroxysteroids—Corticoids containing OH groups on the molecule.

17-Hydroxysteroids—Steroids containing the OH groups at the 17 position.

Total 17 Hydroxysteroids—A term used to signify the urinary measurement of all 17-OH containing steroids following the hydrolysis of the conjugates.

IV Hydrocortisone—Hydrocortisone sodium succinate or hydrocortisone phosphate (as hydrocortisone 21—phosphate, disodium salt).

Juxtaglomerular Apparatus—A group of cells situated at the afferent arteriolar inlet of each glomerulus. Thought to be the source of renin.

∝-Ketol Side Chain—The 20-keto, 21-hydroxy group, is a side chain possessed by all active corticosteroids. It has reducing properties used in the chemical determination of corticosteroids.

17-Ketogenic Steroids (17-KGS)—Steroids measured in the urine derived from substances which can be converted to 17-ketosteroids.

17-Ketosteroids—All steroids appearing in urine with a keto group in the 17 position. This is a term formerly used to denote androgenic steroids. The term is no longer an accurate measure of androgenicity.

Macula Densa—A ridge of cells in the juxtaglomerular apparatus which is thought to sense stretch of the arteriole and thus control release of renin from the juxtaglomerular apparatus. The macula densa may also be responsive directly to sodium concentration in the distal tubule.

Metabolic Clearance Rate (MCR)—The rate at which a steroid is cleared from the plasma. It is usually expressed in liters per hour and is a measure of the metabolism of a steroid. For most steroids this occurs almost completely in the liver.

Medulla—The inner zone of the adrenal gland. The location for both production and secretion of epinephrine and norepinephrine.

Metyrapone (Metopirone)—A substance which inhibits hydroxylation on the 11-position of the adrenal steroid molecule. It is used to test for ability of the pituitary to secrete ACTH and in the differential diagnosis of Cushing's Syndrome.

Mineralocorticoids—All steroids possessing the ability to stimulate the reabsorption of sodium in the distal tubule in exchange for potassium and hydrogen ion.

Nelson's Syndrome—A syndrome described by Dr. D. H. Nelson in 1959, due to progressive enlargement of the pituitary gland and excessive excretion of ACTH and MSH in patients treated for Cushing's Syndrome with bilateral adrenalectomy.

Neutral Steroids—Those steroids which do not possess a phenolic hydroxy group in the A-ring and are therefore neutral in solution.

11-Oxysteroids (OXO) or 11-Oxygenated Steroids—Those steroids possessing an oxygen atom either as a ketol or a hydroxy group in the 11-position. Since the adrenal cortex alone possesses the ability to hydroxylate (or to oxygenate) the position, this is a designation used to stipulate the adrenal cortex as the site of origin of the steroid as opposed to the ovary or the testis which possess little 11-hydroxylase enzyme.

Parenteral hydrocortisone—See IV hydrocortisone.

Porter-Silber Chromagens—A term used for those steroids, cortisol, cortisone and compound S, which possess the 17, 21-dihydroxy-20-ketone group. This group reacts with acid phenylhydrazine to form a yellow compound, the intensity of which is directly proportional to the amount of steroid present. This has long been used as a measure of cortisol in both plasma and urine.

Pregnenetriol—The degredation product of 17-hydroxyprogesterone appearing in excess in the urine in the adrenogenital syndrome and in normal pregnancy.

Progesterone—A steroid produced in large quantities by the adrenal and by the placenta in pregnancy which has a progestational effect.

Renin—A polypeptide produced by the juxtaglomerular apparatus of the kidney which is converted by enzymes in the plasma to angiotensin which then helps control the secretion of aldosterone from the adrenal zona glomerulosa.

Rhythm—Adrenal steroids are secreted and excreted in a rhythmic pattern during a 24-hour period. Several terms describing aspects of this have been used imprecisely and give rise to confusion.

a. ***Circadian***—pertaining to the 24-hour periodicity of secretion. The most common term used.
b. ***Diurnal***—pertaining to that part of the cycle occurring during the day. Often used instead of circadian.
c. ***Nocturnal***—the pattern of plasma and urine steroid secretion occurring through the night.
d. ***Nyctohemeral***—an alternative to circadian referring to both day and night rhythm.

Secretion Rate—The rate at which a steroid is secreted from its parent gland. It is usually measured by isotope dilution. Its measurement combined with that of the metabolic clearance rate gives the most accurate estimation of production and disposal of steroids.

Spironolactone—A synthetic substance which inhibits the action of aldosterone on the distal tubule of the nephron by competitive inhibition.

Steroid—Those compounds containing a four-ring structure, the cyclopentano-perhydrophenanthrene nucleus.

Synthetic Steroids—Any steroid produced biosynthetically or chemically outside the mammalian body.

Testosterone—The most potent androgenic substance produced in large amounts by the testis but also in very small amounts by the ovary, the adrenal and in peripheral tissues, particularly muscle and liver by conversion of adrenal precursors. In excess it produces hirsutism and virilism.

Tetrahydrocortisol—The urinary metabolite produced in the liver by hydroxylation of the $\triangle^{4\text{-}3}$ ketone group of cortisol.

Tetrahydrocortisone—The urinary metabolite produced in the liver by hydroxylation of the $\triangle^{4\text{-}3}$ ketone group of cortisone.

Transcortin—See CBG.

Urinary Steroids—A term applied to all steroids appearing in the urine. They are metabolically inactive although a very small fraction of free active steroids is excreted.

Urinary Conjugates—See conjugates.

Venography (Adrenal venography)—A radiographic technique whereby radiographic contrast material is infused retrogradely through the veins around the adrenal gland.

Virilism—A state of excess androgenicity in the female or the early appearance of puberty in the male. Hirsutism is one aspect of virilism.

X-Zone—A term applied to the outer zone of the adrenal cortex in mice. Not to be confused with the fetal zone in humans.

Zimmerman Reaction—The classic reaction for measurement of 17-ketosteroids in the urine with sodium metadinitrobenzene first described in 1936 by Dr. Wilhelm Zimmermann.

Zona Glomerulosa—The outer zone of the adrenal cortex which predominantly produces aldosterone.

Zona Fasciculata—The middle zone of the adrenal cortex associated with the production of cortisol and other adrenal steroids.

Zona Reticularis—The inner zone of the adrenal cortex associated with functions similar to that of zona fasciculata.

Acknowledgements

Figure 1
Dr. J. C. Houston, Dean of Medicine, Guy's Hospital, London Bridge, SE19RT, England.

Figure 5
Dr. W. E. Hassan, Jr., Director, Peter Bent Brigham Hospital, Boston, MA.

Figures 7 and 8
Dr. J. W. Conn, Professor of Medicine, University of Michigan Medical Center, Ann Arbor, MI.

Figure 9
Adapted from The Adrenals, Peter H. Forsham, in *Textbook of Endocrinology*, Ed. R. W. William, W. B. Saunders Company, 1968.

Figures 11, 12, 14, 17, and 40
D. Slotton, Medical Illustrator, Los Angeles, CA.

Figures 13a, b, c, 15, 80a, b, 82, and 86
Dr. F. W. Turner, Professor of Radiology and Medicine, USC School of Medicine, Los Angeles, CA.

Figures 16 and 85
Dr. N. W. Warner, Professor and Chairman, Department of Pathology, U.S.C. School of Medicine, Los Angeles, CA.

Figures 21a, b
Dr. B. W. Harding, Professor of Biochemistry and Medicine, U.S.C. School of Medicine, Los Angeles, CA.

Figure 36
Adapted from D. T. Krieger, Mount Sinai School of Medicine, in Hospital Practice, September, 1971.

Figure 38
Adapted from Weitzman et al., J. C. Endocrin, *33*:14, 1971.

Figure 43
Dr. Richard Horton, Chief, Section of Endocrinology, U.S.C. School of Medicine, Los Angeles, CA.

Figure 45
Adapted from August, Nelson and Thorn, J. Clin. Invest. *37*:1549, 1958.

Figures 49, 50, 54, 55, 56, 57, 58, 59, 60, 61, 62, 66, 67, 68, 69, 70, 71a, b, 73, 75a, b, c, d, 76, 77, 78, 83
Los Angeles County/Univ. Southern California (LAC/USC) Medical Center, Los Angeles, CA.

Figures 87 and 88
Dr. Roger Terry, Professor of Pathology, U.S.C. School of Medicine, Los Angeles, CA.

Figures 91, 92, 93 94a, b, c
Dr. D. F. Frasier, Professor of Pediatrics and Dr. R. Robert Penny, Assistant Professor of Pediatics, U.S.C. School of Medicine, Los Angeles, CA.